NAOMI SEDDON

Milk *and* Margaritas

We acknowledge the Traditional Custodians of country throughout Australia and their connections to lands, waters and communities. We pay our respect to Elders past and present and extend that respect to all Aboriginal and Torres Straight Islander peoples today. We honor these people, their stories and culture.

Some of the people in this book have had their names changed to protect their identities.

First published 2021.
Copyright © Naomi Seddon 2021
ISBN: 978-168564254-9

To my daughters Savannah & Adaline.
You are the best part of me.
I would do it all again 1000 times over for you.

CONTENTS

Part 1

NAVIGATING HEALTH ISSUES AND HEARTACHE ON THE CAREER LADDER

Part 2

WOMEN'S HEALTH ISSUES IN THE WORKPLACE - A HANDBOOK FOR A MODERN WORLD

Milk and Margaritas

One woman's story of health, heartbreak and
career that speaks on behalf of all women,
carrying a critical message for workplaces
across the globe

Foreword

FOREWORD BY JAS RAWLINSON

I may not know your story, or what life experiences have led you to hold this book within your hands, but I can hand-on-heart tell you that Naomi's story – and the insights within *Milk and Margaritas* – will challenge, inspire, and move you in unexpected and surprising ways.

Throughout my many years of working with women as a book coach and freelance journalist, I've often advocated for awareness around the debilitating physical and mental impacts of issues such as endometriosis, PMDD and PCOS, and the need for more understanding and support. Likewise, as a friend to many women who struggle with these conditions, I've rallied to help break the stigma around what they are experiencing, often fighting alongside them in the push for better medical, psychological and financial support. Yet, it was not until I met Naomi and heard her vision for this book, that I connected the dots between workplace gender equality and women's experiences with these very issues.

Like many working women, I've experienced my fair share of, 'keep this pain to yourself and don't ask for help' moments. Moments where I was more concerned about being seen as capable and productive to my employers than taking time off to deal with a biological reality I had no control over. As a result, I internalized the belief that female-exclusive health conditions, like agonizing periods, polycystic ovarian syndrome, fertility struggles, and menopause were health challenges that we, as women, needed to deal with outside of the workplace and keep to ourselves, at best hoping for a little bit of sympathy from our bosses. I'm also somewhat embarrassed to admit that I was one of those people who didn't really believe that gender inequality was an issue still prevalent in Western workplaces.

Milk and Margaritas quickly destroyed those beliefs that I'd held for so long.

As Naomi and I began to work together, and I learned more about her own journey and the research that she had been championing for so many years, I came to realize that there were still many ways in which women were being held back from meaningful and sustainable employment, for no reason other than their own biology and the attitude of their workplaces.

You might be surprised to know that, during the writing of this book, Naomi struggled severely with her own health and chronic pain conditions. At times her endometriosis and pain flare-ups were so severe that she struggled to get words onto paper. Even so, she never gave up. This book was a labor of love, and she was committed to finishing it. Not just for herself, but for you: the dear reader who now holds this book within your hands.

It was an honor to work with Naomi on Milk and Margaritas and I'm grateful our paths were so beautifully brought together on such an important project. It is a book that will challenge you to rethink your own beliefs, and one that will encourage employers to use their positions of power and leadership to create change. Equally important, it is a powerful source of support and validation for working women. A collection of words that say, I see you, your pain is valid, and you're not alone'.

Well-researched, captivating, and filled with vulnerable storytelling, Milk and Margaritas is a groundbreaking, must-read book for all workplaces, management teams, and those in positions of leadership. As Naomi herself shares: "Unless we start having conversations within our workplaces to find out what the needs of our female employees are, and unless we start leading with empathy and empowering women to find better ways to thrive and succeed at work, then the goal of equality that so many amazing women before us have fought so hard to achieve, is just not going to be within our reach."

JAS RAWLINSON,
- Best-selling author, award-nominated book coach and resilience speaker

FOREWORD BY DONNA CICCIA

We have all heard the saying, 'life is precious' – there comes a time in our lives that this statement rings true and we finally have clarity and understanding of the depth of its meaning.

For myself, the first time this statement's true meaning came was at the birth of my son – when I was holding him in my arms for the very first time. The next time was when we lost our second and deeply longed-for child through miscarriage, after our first of many subsequent attempts at IVF. You see, I too have endometriosis just like Naomi. My diagnosis and loss led me to being a founder of Endometriosis Australia, an organization that is dear to my heart and which I often refer to as the second child I could never have. This is how Naomi and I crossed paths, and while we have some similar experiences with this horrid disease, our lives have taken different directions to raise awareness.

There are moments in our lives when all we can do is put one foot in front of the other to get through the day. Many other times, our lives can be about reflecting and learning from those experiences, good and bad, and if the opportunity presents itself, we can use this knowledge and share it with others. Naomi brings all these elements together in her book to empower the reader with her lived experience and expertise.

It would be remiss of me to put down words on paper without speaking out and explaining what endometriosis is and why it is important to continue to shine a light on a disease that still too many live with in silence.

Endometriosis is a disease that can have wide and far-reaching effects on someone's life. It is a disease where cells similar to the lining of the uterus grow elsewhere in the body. It is commonly found around the pelvis, but has been found as far away as the lungs and the brain. Each person's experience with this disease varies widely. Some have fertility issues, some may have pain and fatigue issues and others have little or no symptoms at all. Endometriosis affects one in nine women, and those that identify as gender diverse in

Australia[1], and the latest research indicates it costs the Australian economy $9.7 billion annually[2] through direct and indirect costs.

I believe empowering ourselves and those around us with knowledge will ultimately help us reach our potential. Naomi's book does this in spades. Together we can all be a part of the solution.

DONNA CICCIA,
- *Director & Co-Founder, Endometriosis Australia*

FOREWORD BY BEVAN SLATTERY

In 2015 I was flying back to Australia from the US after spending time on one of my latest startups - Megaport. It was a really hectic time - made even more hectic because of a promise I had made to my young family years earlier. I would always be home for the weekend, no matter where I was around the world. So it was a Thursday night flight out of LA. I had settled into my preferred aisle seat when I noticed this smiling bundle of hope next to me. When you meet lots of people, sometimes you just know someone is inherently kind and optimistic. It's in the eyes and the smile. They almost always smile and they acknowledge you and make you feel welcome... relaxed in fact. That person of course was Naomi.

The stories Naomi shared on that flight were at times breathtaking, horrifying, extraordinary, beautiful, empowering, saddening but ultimately inspiring. Inspiring because despite so much happening to one person, with such adversity here was this woman who was not thinking of herself but thinking of how to help others. Focused on how to empower others. I went home and always spoke about Naomi to others and what an inspiring story she had.

I asked Naomi to come and meet my team at Megaport, which she did the next day and she started assisting the team with our U.S.

1. Rowlands I, Abbott J, Montgomery G, Hockey R, Rogers P, Mishra G. Prevalence and incidence of endometriosis in Australian women: A data linkage cohort study. Br J Obstet Gynaecol 2021; 128(4): 657-65.

2. Armour M, Lawson K, Wood A, Smith CA, Abbott J. The cost of illness and economic burden of endometriosis and chronic pelvic pain in Australia: A national online survey. PLoS ONE 2019; 14(10): e0223316.

expansion. A year later I reached out to Naomi again to help Megaport professionally on a legal matter and it was at that time I knew that I needed to give that spirit and commitment to create positive change, a platform. There are too few women on public company Boards and part of that problem is that too few businesses give women their first Board seat. So I later asked if she would join Megaport as a Director - "Absolutely, I'd be honoured" was the answer and we haven't looked back. Today Naomi is the cultural champion for diversity and inclusiveness on the Megaport Board and beyond.

We all have those sliding door moments. It is truly remarkable how often the greatest change comes from the most simple beginnings. A chance seat on a plane and Naomi's courage to strike up a conversation with the random person right next to her. Oh yes... Courage, "the ability to do something that frightens one: bravery." That's another word to describe Naomi.

How someone possesses so much courage with equal amounts of empathy is inspiring and something we need to celebrate and share. *Milk and Margaritas*? You bet and I'll raise my glass to that.

BEVAN SLATTERY,
- Founder of SUB.CO, Cloudscene, Superloop, Megaport, NEXTDC and Co-Founder PIPE Networks

Introduction

Women's health is a worldwide problem in workplaces and is a major contributor to the 'gender gap'. Gender inequality is measured on the World Economic Forum's Global Gender Gap Index. At the current rate, at which gender inequality is being reduced, especially due to the impacts of COVID-19, it will take 135.6 years[3] to close the gap completely. That means that it is unlikely that there are many people alive today who will see significant change within their lifetime. It also means that my daughters and for those of you who also have daughters – probably theirs as well – will likely never see it in their lifetimes either. To me, that is simply unacceptable. We MUST find a way to do better!

As a result of the global pandemic, the situation has worsened. Women have withdrawn from the workforce at alarming rates and studies indicate that many will not return. Companies cannot afford to lose women leaders. Research has shown that company profits and share performance can be close to fifty percent higher when women are well-represented[4]. It also has a direct cost to the economy, as it is estimated that closing the gap on gender equality could increase global GDP by up to $20 trillion dollars.

Women also dominate the global economy when it comes to consumer spending at approximately $20 trillion annually. That figure could climb as high as $28 trillion in the next five years, yet amazingly so many companies continue to fail to recognize this. The beauty and luxury goods industries for example, are dominated by men trying to sell to women. According to the Fortune 500 and S&P 500 companies of 2020, only thirty-seven are led by women, and only one of these is in the beauty industry. Why does this matter? According to a 2016 paper, published by The National Bureau of Economic Research, it shows that having a female CEO overseeing

---

3. https://www.weforum.org/reports/global-gender-gap-report-2021/digest/

4. https://www.mckinsey.com/featured-insights/diversity-and-inclusion/diversity-wins-how-inclusion-matters

a workforce of at least twenty percent women, would increase sales per employee by one percent, and for almost every single company, its sales function is its most important area of operations. After all, without sales, a company has no business.

However, as the number of women in the workforce is declining, it is more important than ever before to find better ways to support women at work. Until we start recognizing that women are fundamentally different to men and therefore our experiences and needs at work are different, we cannot hope to close the gap on gender equality.

The statistics clearly show us that almost every single woman will at some point in their life experience health issues related to menstruation, fertility, pregnancy loss, menopause, endometriosis, or another gynecological condition. Literally, almost every single woman! So, why do we continue to impose requirements in the workplace and implement policies and practices that we expect should suit every employee? Why does there remain such a stigma attached to these issues? This is so detrimental, and a fear exists amongst women that discussing their health issues is in some way showing a perceived weakness, and therefore there is an overwhelming, general unwillingness to accept that these very real problems are issues that should be discussed and supported in the workplace. I think there are a number of reasons for this, and as I detail throughout this book, there are some things that every single one of us can do to change the narrative around this vitally important issue.

There is a significant amount of evidence to demonstrate the link between productivity and wellness. I would like to demonstrate to all employers, that not only will finding better ways to support your female employees make you employers of choice, better employers, and empathetic employers and leaders, but it will also improve the bottom line. The research shows us time and again that employers who look after their employees end up with happier, more productive employees with lower turnover and recruitment costs, and this just skims the surface of the benefits that an organization will see as a result of prioritizing employee mental health and wellness.

As a woman who has worked her way to the top, while suffering from more than her fair share of health issues, I have learnt a lot of hard lessons along the way. It is my sincere belief that unless we start having conversations within our workplaces to find out what the needs of our female employees are, unless we start leading with empathy and empowering women to find better ways to thrive and succeed at work, then that goal of equality that so many amazing women before me have fought so hard to achieve, is just not going to be within our reach.

It is my hope that you will join me on this journey, and afterwards, help to start a movement by having discussions within your own organizations about these issues and demanding change through action and advocacy. If we all just do one small thing each day to lead us in the right direction, it is progress, and one step forward is all we need to make change happen. I am here to assist and guide you, and I am cheering you all on from my corner of the world, as you take that first step to raise these issues within your own communities, families, and organizations.

PART 1

Navigating health issues and heartache on the career ladder

My Story

It is a beautiful sunny day here in Los Angeles, as most days are here, and I am wondering where to begin to tell you 'my' story. I feel so blessed to be sitting here on my lounge chair, enjoying the afternoon sun under the shade of the hundred-year-old palm tree that sits in the corner of my backyard. My journey to get here was far from easy. I have learnt a lot along the way about humans. Lessons about life, love, sacrifice, commitment, compassion, empathy, culture, diversity, the career ladder. I feel compelled to share my story with you in the hope that by doing so, I might be able to start discussions within more workplaces, amongst more managers, executives and employees and in more board meetings, about some of these issues, to get a better deal for all female employees.

Over the years, almost every time I have told someone my story, inevitably they have said, "You've got to write a book". It took me a while to get to the point where I have felt able to share my story so publicly, but I always knew it was something I wanted to do. I believe my experiences and the things I have learnt along the way as a result, have the potential to change workplaces, to change the way we think about employees, and ultimately to move far closer towards achieving equality in the workplace than we ever have before. I am also hopeful that by sharing my insights, it might resonate with leaders who will want to implement positive changes within their own organizations.

I recently watched the Prince Harry and Oprah production, *The Me You Can't See*, and one of the things that Prince Harry said was, "Telling stories is healing for the person sharing, healing for those receiving the message also, as they know that they are not alone, and stories are also what are needed to start discussions about making positive changes." I wholeheartedly believe this too, and if you haven't watched the series, then I highly recommend it because, although it was focused on mental health issues generally, so much of what the experts said throughout the program is equally applicable here.

No one knows the silent struggles another person may be facing in this unpredictable life; none of us know if something similar might happen to us. This is why it is crucial to provide employees with the resources, information and support they need to feel comfortable enough to speak up, take time out and to ask for help when needed. While I certainly did go through a lot more than most other people experience by the age of thirty-five, I also know without a doubt that many of the experiences I have had in my life are definitely not unique. Many women go through similar experiences as well and that is at the heart of why I wanted to write this book. So, thank you for taking this journey with me.

*

I had what some might call a turbulent start in life. My mother had been sheltered throughout her life and was a very immature twenty-one-year-old, with little life experience and unfortunately, she fell for the charm of a con artist. She fell pregnant to a man sixteen years her senior – a man who ultimately ended up treating my mother and I VERY badly! They married shortly after, as back then, when 'accidents' happened, it seemed the respectable thing to do. She was also fearful of bringing up a daughter on her own, although finally she received so much support from her family. My mother finally left my father when I was about two-and-a-half years of age and we went to live with my nana.

For all of the pain I experienced because of my 'father', my nana made up for it in spades. She was, and still is to this day, the most special human I have ever had the privilege of knowing, and everything that I am today I owe to her. She taught me so many life lessons, including that you can achieve anything with enough passion, hard work, and dedication. She also taught me the importance of love, compassion, empathy and above all, the importance of showing kindness to others. One of her favorite things to say was, "Don't ever judge another person until you walk in their shoes." And honestly, that really is so applicable to the things I am going to share with you throughout this book.

As young children, we often see people or events through rose-colored glasses, so as an adult I now try to look back on my nana's life to find the faults or flaws in her character. But honestly, there really aren't many at all in my eyes. She was the closest thing to perfection to me. She had more faith and conviction than I have ever seen in another person, and it never wavered. She was highly intelligent, extremely loving, and full of compassion and empathy for others. She never had very much materially, but had a strong faith in God and truly lived the life of authentic Christianity, trusting God for his provisions in her life.

She demonstrated real contentment and was never envious of others. If she saw someone in need she would always, always help. Many a night we would turn up to Nana's house and my mother and Nana would whip up some meal for us. She loved her children and grandchildren, and her greatest delight was visits from us all. It wasn't just her generosity towards family though. Nana was known to help anyone in need, all the time. She would have given the shirt off her own back if it would have helped someone. She was just that kind of person. I will never stop missing her, but I am forever blessed to have called her my nana and to have been able to spend so much time with her. She was my best friend, and I am so thankful to be able to honor her memory here in this way.

My mother remarried when I was almost five, and as a result, I have two wonderful brothers I am very close to. My mother and father made sure that we all had many special experiences and celebrations as a family; vacations, Christmas, Easter, special outings to the zoo etc. and they were happy times as a family. They both worked hard, but like all young couples who are starting out, it was never easy and there were always financial stresses. I was determined from a young age to create a life for myself, so that I could be financially independent. I never wanted to have to experience sleepless nights worrying about how I was going to pay the bills.

My nana was my biggest supporter. She would say to me often, "Naomi, reach for the stars" and "All you need is faith the size of a mustard seed to move a mountain". She even bought a silver locket for me which housed one tiny mustard seed and I wore that locket all through my final year of high school exams, when I was desperately trying to achieve a high enough final score to obtain a place in law school. Just knowing that little mustard seed was around my neck, as I dedicated myself to my studies during those years, helped me to keep going and strive forward and upwards towards my dreams.

Having just one person who is in your corner, one person who wants you to succeed, is all that any person needs and it can literally change the course of a person's life. I have tried to remember this throughout my working life too, because it is equally applicable to us as we get older as it is to a young child. Ultimately, as a result of hard work, determination and support, as well as a few setbacks, I did get into law school. I finished my degree and I have had many achievements since then that have led me to where I find myself today.

I finished high school in 1999 and at the time I thought my dreams were over, as I missed out by just .05 marks on obtaining a place at Melbourne Monash University, where I had wanted to do my law degree. I had my heart set on Monash after completing a wonderful internship with Judge Hasset at the County Court, who when I asked for his advice on where I should study law told me, "You go to Melbourne for the name. You go to Monash if you want a good education". From that day onwards, I was set on obtaining my degree there. I was also sure that based on my marks I would receive a second-round offer at Monash, but it ultimately wasn't meant to be and instead I obtained an offer from the Australian National University in Canberra.

ANU was my second choice, because at the time, I had wanted to study political law, as I had always thought I might end up going into politics one day. Although that is not a path I have ended up taking, my work has always involved strong connections to government. I have advised on complex foreign government legal issues, worked with a number of government trade departments and have presented at many government events over the years on market entry, trade and investment, and other international legal topics including my passion – women's health issues in the workplace.

In any event, as I had waited until the final offer stages to accept the place at ANU while I had been holding out hope of a second round offer at Monash, I ended up having twenty-four hours to get up to Canberra from Melbourne to enroll, in order to accept my place there. As flights were very expensive back then, especially for an eighteen-year-old, I managed to get an overnight bus to Canberra. The bus left from the Melbourne CBD and arrived in Canberra at 5am. Because it had been such a last-minute arrangement, there really wasn't any time to make a solid plan or to really think through what I was going to do when I arrived so early in the morning.

Needless to say, the bus station was empty within a few minutes of arriving. The other passengers quickly collected their luggage and scurried away into the cold night air. The station was deserted. I went and found a seat to park myself at in a lighted area where I decided to read a book and wait until a coffee shop opened, so that I could get some breakfast before I headed off in the direction of ANU. I had planned to spend the day enrolling, purchasing the required textbooks on my book list, and touring the campus before taking the same overnight bus back to Melbourne that evening. I would then have two weeks before I would need to get back to Canberra to commence classes. There was a lot to plan in two weeks, but I needed to head back to Melbourne to settle things there first, before I could relocate for the next four years to complete my degree. I was full of excitement. This was what I had been working hard for and it was to be the start of the rest of my life.

I will never know what life at ANU would have been like though, because I never did make it there. I haven't thought of this for many years and just writing this now, I can almost feel once again what it was like to be there in that moment, so terrified and isolated. As I sat alone at that station reading my book, all of a sudden, I became aware of someone's presence. I don't know where he came from or how long he had been watching me, but suddenly a man was seated right next to me, far too close for comfort. I will never forget his eyes. They were large and bloodshot, and he had a crazed look about him. He leaned into me a few inches from my face and started asking me to come home with him.

I recoiled and attempted to move away from the man as quickly as I could, but he was unrelenting. He came at me with displeasure at my refusal and demanded that I would be coming with him. He tried to grab me and told me that there was no one around who could save me. I was all alone. I knew that he was much bigger and stronger than me and that if he did grab me, I would find it difficult to break free. In a split second I made a decision. I ran as fast as my feet could carry me towards the rest rooms. I knew that if I went in there, he would be sure to follow me and then I would be trapped, but I also knew that they were situated around a corner and that if I was fast enough, I just might have a chance to execute my on-the-fly plan.

I ducked as the man launched his body towards me and I ran. I pushed the door to the women's restroom open with great force so that it was still swinging while I launched myself into the men's restroom door, being careful to stop the door from swinging as I stood against it on the other side. When I heard the man running after me into the women's restroom, I could hear him pushing the doors of the toilet stalls open, I then made my escape. I ran out of the men's restroom and out into the night as fast as my legs would carry me and I never looked back.

I don't know how long I was running for or how far I actually ran, but I never stopped praying and I didn't stop until the first light of sunrise peeked through the morning clouds and the city started waking, ready for the day ahead. I was frightened and confused and had no idea where I was or where I should go. I managed to find a police station and I filed a report. I then contacted my parents and arrangements were made for me to fly home right away.

When I returned to Melbourne I was in a bad state. I was in shock after what had happened to me, and I was scared! Had it just been that one incident that occurred though, I may have still ended up at ANU. Maybe, I don't know. However, less than a week later, I was traveling home from work one day and I was attacked again. This time at Boronia train station in Melbourne. It was about four pm in the afternoon this time, and I was standing on the station platform minding my own business when four gang members came up to me and started spitting on me and screaming abuse at me. One of them pulled a knife out, demanding my purse. Luckily, another passenger pushed the emergency button on the platform and tried to assist until the police arrived. Once again, I found myself sitting at a police station that evening filing a report, this time thankfully, with my dad by my side.

After the second attack, I was understandably a mess. I was in no fit condition to be moving to another state on my own to embark on a law degree. I just couldn't do it. So, I made the decision to defer my place and take a gap year. It was one of the best decisions I have ever made. In that year, I gained life and work experience. I travelled and spent time with family and friends. I also allowed myself the time that I needed to heal. There were points during that year that I wondered whether I would ever end up obtaining my law degree, but eventually, I had a plan that I intended to stick to and I finally knew that somehow, I would make it happen once the time was right.

I am a huge advocate for young people taking a gap year. I really do think that it gives you a much better frame of mind entering the difficult years of study that lie ahead. However, I also know the impact that experiences like that can have on a person's mental health, and how difficult it is to get up again and keep moving forward. These are the types of events that so many women experience every single day in every country in the world and for many of these women, they never recover and are never the same.

This is another reason why we simply must try to do better to protect and support female employees in the workplace because experiences of sexual harassment, assault and abuse happen every day, both generally within society and within workplaces everywhere. It is estimated that approximately eighty-one percent of women globally have experienced some form of sexual harassment – approximately half of all cases occurring at work – and most never report it. It is also important to note that one in three women globally are also estimated to experience violence in their lifetimes.

After my gap year, I wasn't sure if I was ready to go back and I still felt apprehension about being so far away from my family in Canberra, but that is where I gained my place and where I would have to go if I was going to fulfill my dream, so I was conflicted. It was the week before enrollment, and I didn't know what to do. As much as I wanted to study law, ultimately, I just knew that ANU wasn't for me. It was all still too raw, and I needed the love and support of my family and friends around me at that time. I decided to withdraw and so again I ended up in the week of enrollment with no university place.

Fortunately though, my mother, who is a teacher, happened to have a child in her class that year whose mother was one of the admissions coordinators at Deakin University. I had achieved well over the required score to obtain a place in law at that university and so, after hearing about what had happened to me, they kindly agreed to offer me a last-minute place. I started my law degree at Deakin a week later and graduated with my law degree in November 2005, with my family by my side, including my nana. It was one of the happiest days of my life and I am so grateful that she was there to share in my achievement.

I never did forget about my desire to study at Monash though, and so a few years after I obtained my law degree, I decided to go back to study. I obtained my Master of Laws from Monash University in 2011. Obtaining that degree was the start of my journey into international law. So, whenever a door closes on you, don't ever think that the door won't open for you again. Sometimes you do get another opportunity, so be ready when it does!

Turning Lemons into Margaritas

In 2010, I was Legal Counsel at the Australian Industry Group in Melbourne. I loved my job. My team and I had a wonderful boss, but something happened to me that year that would change the course of my life forever. Something that at the time was so awful that I could never have imagined the incredible opportunities that would eventually come my way as a result – I really did turn lemons, and bad lemons at that, into margaritas.

After finishing my law degree, I went on a Contiki Tour of Europe in the summer of 2006. I met some wonderful people on that tour who I still call some of my closest friends today. We had planned a trip in 2010 to all meet up in the U.S. again and so in March I headed off to meet my friends in San Francisco, where we would start our road trip of the U.S. together. We drove to L.A. first and then went on to Las Vegas. It was my first time in the city of lights, which has become one of my favorite cities in the world. I had my thirtieth birthday in Vegas and even got married there on my birthday in 2015. But this story is not about my husband. This story is about what happened to me that caused me to relocate to the U.S. Ultimately, I did end up meeting my wonderful husband, Dave, in San Francisco, but that is much later in my story.

My friends and I had an amazing time in Vegas. I have now visited the city about thirty times, but nothing compares to seeing Vegas for the first time. There is something magical about the city. There are a lot of people who dislike Vegas, but there is so much to do in this city that I don't think you could possibly hope to discover it all, even if you stayed for a year. I am not a gambler at all. In fact, I don't think I have ever spent more than twenty dollars on a slot machine in Vegas, but the thing that I love about Vegas is the diversity and eclectic nature of the city. It is a place where people from all walks of life can come and experience some fun – whatever that might look like, as there are many different types of fun to be had in the city of lights. It really is a place where you can spend a few days in a different world that is far removed from the reality of most people's lives, and I love that! This is also why so many major conferences are held in the city each year. It is a great place to host clients or hold meetings because there is no shortage of hotels, bars and restaurants. So, I generally try to get to Vegas at least a couple of times a year for a few days.

On my first trip to Vegas in 2010 though, I was just trying to soak it all in – the glitz and glam of this fascinating city with some of my favorite people on this earth. It was an amazing trip and I still think back to my time with my friends on both the Contiki tour and then the subsequent trip around the U.S. as one of my happiest life memories. Something happened on that trip though that would change the course of my life forever. I met someone at a bar at the MGM Grand. Let's just call him Rick. The man that I met was someone that seemed perfect, too good to be true... and he was! He was British and was in Vegas for the week with some of his friends. We instantly connected and over the course of the next four days we were inseparable. Rick went everywhere with us for the next few days, and I too met some of the friends he had travelled to Vegas with. We had such an instant connection. He was like no one I had ever met before, and I fell instantly in love.

By the end of the trip, we reluctantly parted with an agreement that Rick would come to Melbourne soon to visit me. I had a few more weeks with my friends in the U.S. and then Mexico before returning home to Melbourne. By the time I got home he had already booked a trip to come and see me. Coincidentally, my mother was living in London at the time teaching there for a year, so he also went to meet my mother before I saw him again. During that meeting, Rick told my mother he was going to marry me. She too fell for his charming ways and gave her blessing. Then, six months later, after multiple trips to Australia every few weeks, he did indeed propose with a beautiful ring. Everyone who met Rick fell in love with him and I was the happiest I had ever been. Sadly, it only lasted for a short while. Soon after the engagement, things started to unravel and cracks started to show in his personality, and the events that transpired that year were nothing short of horrific!

Rick had left Melbourne shortly after our engagement to return to the U.K. and he had planned to come back about a month later with his two children. That trip I started to notice a few odd behaviors. There were things I had not seen before. Even though he did live in another country, we had actually spent a lot of time together because he had flown back and forth to Melbourne every two or three weeks during the months that we had been dating. Rick was a Sergeant Major in the British Army. He had told me he had a lot of accrued leave because he had recently completed a fourth deployment to Afghanistan. He also told me he had a lot of savings, which is why he was able to afford the many flights to and from Australia. As it turned out though, a lot of what he had told me turned out to be a total fabrication.

I was starting to feel uncomfortable. I was supposed to be planning a wedding and had agreed to move to the U.K. As he had two young sons from a prior marriage, the only way we could be together was if I agreed to move to the U.K. until they were older. I hold British citizenship as well and I had always wanted to live in London, so when we had discussed it initially, I was happy to agree to move. However, I was starting to have concerns. I was worried that I didn't know Rick well enough, and as my mother had returned to Australia, I was concerned that I would be in the U.K. on my own without any family support if things went wrong. There were cracks appearing daily, including sudden bursts of anger that came out of the blue.

Rick did come to Australia a few weeks later with his two sons though and that trip seemed to go well. His sons were wonderful little boys, and I really enjoyed the time I spent getting to know them. I have two brothers who I love spending time with and so I am used to being around boys. I was excited about becoming a stepmother too, especially to two children who seemed so polite and lovely. I therefore tried to tell myself that maybe I was just feeling nervous and that my concerns were only a case of cold feet. Especially when my family and friends liked him so much.

After the trip, Rick left with his sons with a plan to come back to Melbourne two weeks later, as we had started to plan the wedding and there was a lot to do. We had decided to have our wedding reception at a winery in Red Hill, Victoria. I also wanted to get married in a church and so another reason for his next trip back to Melbourne was to start the marriage classes with the minister of the church.

My mother met Rick a few times in London and like everyone who met him, she loved him like a son. However, looking back now, she admits there were a few things that happened in London that she had found a bit strange. She had tried to meet up at Rick's house to see where he lived, but he always had a reason or excuse as to why he had to meet her at a mutual place. When he screamed abuse at a tuk-tuk driver when he didn't agree with the price of the ride, which seemed so out of character at the time, she didn't really question it too much unfortunately, because Rick was just so charming and he explained the situation away (as he always did) and she dismissed these first warning signs.

Rick returned two weeks later and on the first evening he was back in Melbourne, we had dinner at my mother's house. As the evening went on, we had been having a good time together as a family, although he had been in a rather funny mood all night. As the conversation went on, Rick seemed irritated and there was an aggressive tone to his speech. Suddenly, he started talking about some of his experiences in Afghanistan, during his recent deployment. He was saying terrible things. My mother and I became quite distressed and asked him repeatedly to please stop, due to the graphic detail of events. He also had a sort-of crazed look about him. I didn't know if he was drunk, extremely tired, or mentally unwell, but I definitely felt a sense of fear that night, which I knew was not good. I suggested we call it a night, but I felt sick in my stomach. I expressed this to my mother, and she felt the same concern too. I had to take him home and I didn't want to be near him. I just couldn't believe this was the same man I had spent months getting to know. This man was someone I didn't like and now I wasn't sure what I was going to do.

The next day we went to see the church, meet the minister, and complete our first marriage class. Normally the classes are scheduled once a week, over a month, but the minister had agreed to be flexible in the scheduling because of our situation, so our classes would be held over two weekends with longer days. On the way there, I tried to talk to him about the previous night and how much his comments had upset us. I expressed concern at his comments and suggested that they were extremely inappropriate and very strange, so I asked him whether anything was wrong. Rick was in no better mood though than he had been the previous evening, but this time there was no jetlag or alcohol to blame.

The discussion immediately escalated and he became enraged. By the time we reached the church I was feeling awful about the whole situation and the minister could clearly sense this. In fact, I was starting to wonder if I should be getting married to this man at all. We left the meeting and we got into a terrible argument in the car on the way home. Rick had been rude, angry, and nasty at times during the meeting with the minister. I felt extremely anxious and worried, and I asked him what on earth was going on with him. He flew into a rage. He screamed in my face as I was driving, and he tried to punch the side of my face, only missing, and instead smashing his fist into the window as I ducked the punch, whilst veering the car off the road and into the curb.

I was completely shocked and extremely shaken. I started crying hysterically. I couldn't understand what was happening. How had this man who had been so loving and kind, turned into this monster that I didn't even recognize? I was wondering whether he had some type of mental health condition. Rick's next reaction was also concerning because it was as if someone had flicked a switch. In an instant he turned from rage and violence, to meek and mild. Realizing the implications of what he had done, Rick tried to grab and hug me while apologizing over and over. It was all too late for me though. The first warning signs were one thing, but this was beyond enough for me! My mother, my grandmother and great-grandmother had been victims of abuse at the hands of men and I have always been absolutely 100 percent certain of one thing – I was NEVER, EVER going to let any man raise a hand to me!

I want to pause my story here to talk about this for a moment because I know that some of the women who read this book are going to find this section difficult to read. I know that violence and abuse is something that so many women experience and unfortunately some of you will relate to my story. The World Health Organization estimates that one in three women globally are subjected to either physical and/or sexual intimate partner violence, or non-partner sexual violence in their lifetime – one in three!

That figure is real and it is shocking. Violence can impact every aspect of a person's life. It can impact a person's physical and mental health, play havoc with their reproductive health, and it can also damage personal relationships and cause difficulties for a person at work. Having a good support network during a time like this is absolutely crucial! It can mean the difference between a person suffering depression, anxiety or other mental health issues or not.

Having someone to listen and provide comfort, love and support can literally save a person's life. I also know how difficult it can be to be the victim of abuse and not feel able to leave. I know that for some women they are in extremely difficult situations; situations where there does not seem to be a way out, especially if young children are involved. For those people, my heart breaks for you. I urge you to keep trying to find a way and I pray that you will find the courage, resources and support needed to be able to do so. Sometimes all it takes is to share your story with one person.

While I was experiencing the awful situation I went through, I was Legal Counsel at the Australian Industry Group, and I had an incredible and supportive boss and a wonderful team around me. They immediately jumped in to assist me to feel safe in the workplace. They took action to brief the people that needed to know about the situation, and they took steps to provide me with the support that I needed. I cannot tell you how crucial this was and how much I appreciated the assistance and care that my employer showed me during this time. I have absolutely no doubt it was one of the main reasons why I was able to get through what ended up being an incredibly difficult time in my life.

Demonstrating you are an employer who really cares in situations like this is not just the right thing to do; it places you above those companies that don't invest the resources in their people like this. Employees can be your biggest marketing tool, but they also hold great power to cause damage to a company's reputation and unfortunately people listen to and remember negative stories more than positive ones, so it is important to remember this. Time and again, studies have been conducted that clearly show us that those companies who invest in their people and find ways to support their employees through difficulties have happier, more productive, and loyal employees, which in turn, typically reduces costs and increases profitability. I can tell you that even though many years have passed since I was an employee at Ai Group, I always think back fondly of my time there and I cannot count the number of times that I have recommended the organization to clients, colleagues and friends.

After the incident in the car, I realized that Rick was volatile and unpredictable. I also suspected that he might be suffering from post-traumatic stress disorder from his work in Iraq and Afghanistan and I still believe today that is probably true. However, I was not the right person to try to help him and I wasn't even sure whether that was the issue. I am not a psychologist after all and so I was not about to marry a man that was exhibiting the types of behaviors and violence that I had witnessed, until I could be confident that he had a clear understanding that what he had done was wrong, that he needed help and then actually took steps to obtain that help.

I would be there to support Rick through that process, but I was not prepared to proceed to marriage until I could be sure that he was willing to get the help he needed. At first, he said that he understood how I felt and agreed to my terms, but this didn't last long. Ultimately, he ended exhibiting extremely aggressive and abusive behaviors again over the following few weeks and decided against getting the help he needed. Rick also said he refused to accept my decision and demanded that we proceed with the marriage, as I had originally promised to. He became manic and almost desperate. As a result, I realized I had no option but to end the relationship for good. However, from there, the situation escalated, and I had no idea what a horror my life would turn into for the next twelve months.

Over the course of the following year, Rick continued to harass me. He maxed out my credit cards, cleaned out my bank account, sent texts, emails and letters to family, friends, and clients, which not only contained complete lies and abusive language, but clearly demonstrated just how unwell he really was. Rick was completely unrelenting and every single day I would wake up or return home holding my breath to see what new terror he would have in store for me that day. There were days when I would return home to find packages of disgusting items at my doorstep. I received hundreds of phone calls from plastic surgeons, doctors, dentists, and other medical providers that he had contacted pretending to be me and asking them to assist with my obesity or deformities for example.

There were phone calls, emails, letters, packages – hundreds and hundreds of them. Rick also emailed a number of my close friends to tell them that I had slept with their husbands – all complete lies and all calculated to cause me as much stress, humiliation and heartache as possible. He was literally determined to ruin my life in whatever way he could, and he told me this on many occasions in the hundreds of emails he sent me each week. This went on and on and on for months, until I could not take it any longer.

Fortunately, my best friend Sharon is a family lawyer, and she was able to assist me. Something I probably should have done sooner, but I didn't want to have to involve any of my friends and family and I was honestly terrified of him by this point. However, with Sharon's help, I was finally able to obtain a five-year intervention order against Rick, something I understand is incredibly difficult to obtain. Sharon tells me that a twelve-month order is typical in these types of situations, but after reviewing all of the evidence, the Court was so outraged at the extent of the abuse and harassment that he had inflicted upon me during those months that it determined an extended order was appropriate.

His harassment also didn't just end with me. Rick also threatened members of my family as well, which is why I did not want to have to involve them further. Unfortunately, however, my relief at obtaining the intervention order was short-lived, as it was not enough to deter him. In fact, it actually made him behave worse and the difficulty that I faced was that he was in the UK and I was in Australia. In fact, at one point he responded to the Court, confirming he had received the Court Order that had been served upon him in the U.K., but followed on with a tirade of lies about me, including that I was an alcoholic and a drug addict, amongst other things.

You might think I was fortunate that Rick was so far away in the U.K., and in some ways, I was, but it also meant that enforcement of the intervention order was incredibly difficult. What transpired next though was a blessing because it meant that more serious action could be taken. In January 2012, after the intervention order had already been issued, I woke up one morning to literally hundreds of messages on my mobile phone. I then discovered that Rick had put all of my contact details on a prostitution website located in the U.S. He had posted pictures of me, my home address, work address and contact information.

As horrific as this was, it also meant that Rick had now committed a federal offence – stolen identity. He had also threatened to kill me and my family in writing. This meant that we now had the attention of the federal police, so enforcement was much easier to achieve. This set the wheels in motion. I had police assigned to my residence, I had police protection at my work, and I finally felt as though this nightmare might be behind me soon. As crazy as it sounds, I was actually glad that it had happened, as I felt so much safer knowing that there were police watching me, that I actually felt a sense of relief and the stress and anxiety that I had felt for months actually lessened.

In the weeks that followed, the harassment did continue. At the time of issuing the intervention order, the court had directed me to attend sessions with the Victims of Crime Assistance (VCA) program. I had been attending sessions since shortly after the first hearing when the interim order had been issued against him. After the latest issues that I was experiencing, VCA asked me whether I might consider changing my identity. I was determined that I wasn't prepared to do that. I had worked hard to obtain my law degree and build up my career and I wasn't prepared to live without seeing my family. That just wasn't an option for me. They then asked whether I would consider moving overseas for a while and suggested that America might be a good option, because in light of the charges that were pending against Rick, he would not be able to enter America.

I was shocked at first, but by that point I was exhausted as well – physically and mentally, and I desperately wanted all of this to stop for my family's sake as well. I wanted to protect them, and I thought that maybe if I left for a little while, he might at least stop harassing them. I also figured that I could just go until things blew over because the wheels were in motion with the federal police involved now, so I had hope for the first time that Rick might be imprisoned if he continued to harass us all.

So, I made the decision that day in that meeting with VCA that I would go to the U.S., and I would sit the bar exam to become U.S. qualified. I figured that it would take me some time to go through that process anyway and if I passed then maybe I would stay, work and experience life in the U.S. for a while. After all, I certainly needed a fresh start and a break from my current life in Melbourne, given the traumatic year that I had just experienced. I am a person who believes that if something is meant for you then it will work out and I figured that I had nothing to lose by giving it a go. I would take the California bar exam and see what happened.

So, here I was, about to embark on a journey to the U.S. My mother was incredibly sad, but she understood, and having just returned recently from a year in London herself, she knew that living overseas was something that I also wanted to experience, so she accepted my decision. When I told my boss about my decision, he too was fantastic. He understood the reasons for my decision and that a fresh start, even if just for a little while, was what I desperately needed.

I ended up going for an initial six months, first to sit the Multistate Professional Responsibility Examination (MPRE), which is a requirement to practice law in California. The MPRE can be taken before or after the actual bar exam. I elected to take it first, as it is the 'easier' part of the examination process and I figured that it would provide me with a good overview of U.S. law. I passed the MPRE with a ninety-six percent grading, which even though it is nowhere near as extensive as the actual bar exam, made me feel like I was on the right path and with hard work I could probably succeed. By the time I had taken the MPRE, things had settled down and I could probably have gone back home to Australia. However, I was well entrenched in the process and I was loving life as an expat. I was experiencing another part of the world and I had fallen in love again – this time it was a much healthier love – I fell in love with Los Angeles.

It ended up taking me another year to sit the actual California bar exam, which at that time, was a three-day exam. It is now two days. I eventually sat the bar in July 2012, obtained my results in October and ultimately gained admission to the California bar during a swearing in ceremony at the U.S. Consulate in Melbourne. During the entire process, as I sat the exams and completed the various parts of the admissions process, which also involved extensive background checks and applications, my boss at Ai Group let me come and go as I wanted to. I would be gone for a few months in the U.S. to study or sit the various parts of the exam and then I would email him a day or two before I intended to return to Melbourne for another stint.

I returned regularly both for cash and because I could only stay in the U.S. for up to six months at a time on the B visa that I had then. And he would say, "Come right in tomorrow", and away I would go – back to working in my role at Ai Group. I continued like this right up until I permanently relocated to the U.S. The whole process cost me about $90,000 for my flights, the cost of doing the bar preparation courses, sitting the exams, and accommodation in the U.S. during that period. The only reason that I was able to do it was because Ai Group allowed me to come and go during those months, and also due to the generosity of my friend Roland in L.A. Roland was an absolute saint. He is one of those rare, amazingly kind humans.

Roland let me crash on a mattress on his floor for weeks when I was studying for the MPRE. I really do owe both Ai Group and Roland a lot of gratitude because I honestly would never have been able to move to the U.S. if it hadn't been for their flexibility, support, and kindness during my whole journey. To my boss at the time, Peter Nolan, you are an absolute star, an amazing human, and the best industrial relations advisor I have ever seen. I feel honored to have called you a colleague and a friend.

During the period when I was in L.A. studying to sit the actual bar exam, I rented an apartment in Downtown L.A. for two months, because it was cheap! I knew I was going to need to study without distraction and so I locked myself away. I stocked up on food and

I put my head down and my pen to paper. I studied from dawn to dusk. I watched no television for those months, and I went cold turkey on alcohol. I lost eighteen kilograms during those weeks of study. I basically lived on water, coffee, Red Bull and low-fat frozen dinners. I was determined!

I certainly wanted to pass, but what was more important to me was that I was giving it my absolute best shot. I wanted to walk out of the exam on day three and be able to say, "I could not have done anything else because I literally gave it my all". There were so many people who had supported me and given me the tools that I needed to succeed that I was also determined not to let them down. Three months later, I received the results and I found out that I had been one of the lucky people that year who had passed the exam[5]. Passing was honestly a huge bonus at the end of the journey, but it is the achievement that I am most proud of to this day, because of how difficult it was after coming out of such an incredibly traumatic experience.

In the months leading up to the bar exam I was still affected deeply by the events of the previous year, but the stress surrounding my situation with Rick was not yet over. While I was in L.A. studying for the bar, I had woken up one morning to see a troubling email waiting for me in my inbox. It was from the British Military Police, and they were writing to advise me that Rick was in prison. This was a huge relief to me! It also contained an explanation for why the harassment had just suddenly stopped one day, however, the next part of the email made my heart sink to the pit of my stomach.

Rick had not been imprisoned in relation to his crimes against me, rather, he had been convicted of the theft of funds from the British military. As a result, the military investigators were now contacting me about the recovery proceedings that they were in the process of filing against him and potentially me! I later learned that after his conviction, Rick had supposedly agreed to cooperate with the investigation and during that process he had told police investigators that he had given me the stolen funds. In fact, he had been incredibly

---

5. The pass rate for the July 2012 CA bar exam was 54.4% and 12.4% for foreign qualified lawyers.

calculated when concocting his story. Rick told the investigating officers that he had travelled to Australia on twelve occasions, and on each occasion, he had taken in $9,999 in cash with him – just under the mandatory cash reporting amount when entering Australia, which is $10,000.

Because of this, had this been true, Rick would not have had to declare that he was bringing such large amounts of cash into Australia. As a result, they were now coming after me, and once again I was embroiled in an extremely stressful and complex legal mess. I couldn't quite believe that Rick was able to continue to harass me even from behind bars!

This time though, I sprang into action. I was not going to let this man continue to ruin my life, especially when I had tried so hard to forge a new start for myself in the U.S. I immediately contacted a fantastic barrister that I had worked with for many years in Australia, Rob O'Neill. I asked him to take over the handling of the matter for me. I didn't have the energy to attempt to navigate it all myself and besides, I didn't want anything to detract from my focus – studying for and sitting the California bar exam. Don't get me wrong, those months were tough. I often couldn't sleep at night with worry. I felt physically safe for the first time in a long time, but I was also terrified about what was going to happen as a result of this new situation. What if they didn't believe me? What if they came after me for the money that I didn't have?

Ultimately though, I felt secure knowing I was in Rob's extremely capable hands, and I also knew I had the truth on my side because I didn't have even one cent of that money. In fact, as the barrister rightly pointed out to the police, not only did I not have the money, but Rick had also stolen a lot of my own money from me. In the end, after reviewing the ample file that we presented, including the various orders that the Court in Melbourne had issued against him, the police closed their file on me and directed their attention to other areas in seeking recovery of the funds.

I never did learn what happened to Rick because cases involving the military are closed, confidential cases, but I actually don't need or want to know. All that mattered to me was that it was a part of my life, a horrible, horrible part of my life, that was now finally over, and I could move forward. Rob and I still work together to this day, and I am very grateful to him for all the help that he provided to me during those difficult days. As it turns out, Rob has been a part of my story for more than one of the challenging times in my life, as we were also working together on a case in Brisbane years later when I lost my first baby, but more on that later.

When I shared the great news about passing the California bar exam with Peter, my boss at Ai Group, and I told him that I was now ready to move to the U.S., he said he knew someone who was a partner in a law firm in the United States. Peter sat on the ILO Committee in Geneva for Australia and told me that the partner was also on the U.S. Committee. Peter said he knew nothing about the firm, but that the man was lovely and he thought he might be a good contact for me. He sent an email to the partner that said, "One of my best lawyers wants to leave me and she has her heart set on the U.S. She has just taken and passed the California bar exam and so I was wondering whether you might be able to offer her any advice or assistance."

To my surprise, the partner responded and said, "Peter, if that is your recommendation, then I would be pleased to assist her." I flew to San Francisco the next week to meet with him. A week or so later, I went down to L.A. to meet with the team there, as I wanted to be based there. That was Littler, the firm that I still call my professional home today. They made me an offer a few days later and I was on the next flight back to Melbourne where I had my E-3 visa appointment shortly after arriving back there. My visa was issued in about a week, and two days later I was on a flight with my life packed into five suitcases, on my way back to Los Angeles for the beginning of my U.S. adventure. I felt so much excitement and nervous anticipation on that flight. It was the first time I had felt real joy in a very long time. My heart was completely full.

I arrived in Los Angeles on a Friday in October, moved into a very small studio apartment in Santa Monica, and started work at Littler a few days later. I couldn't wait to explore my new world.

L.A. L.A. Land

When I moved to the U.S. I had just reached a stage in my career where I was in a fairly senior role. I was Legal Counsel within my organization, which was the equivalent of a Special Counsel or junior partner level in a firm. However, because I was going to be practicing in a new country an entirely different law applied. One of the things Littler had said to me during the recruitment process was that if I wanted to join the firm, then I would have to essentially start from the bottom again.

They were concerned it would be difficult for me because I was already in a senior role in Australia, but I assured the firm that it didn't bother me. Importantly, I was also prepared to back myself. I know how hard-working I am, and I knew that I would be able to prove myself and progress quickly once I demonstrated results, if that was what I ultimately decided I wanted. However, at that point I wasn't even sure how long I would stay in the U.S. My initial thinking was that I would probably stay a year or maybe two, then go home to Australia. I certainly didn't intend for the U.S to be my permanent home. I also only had a two-year work visa so my expectation at that time was to gain some overseas experience and just see what happened.

About a year after joining the firm and essentially only working on California litigation matters, I realized that I probably wasn't going to be spending my life as a California litigator. I worked hard to learn the litigation landscape, including California law and civil procedure, but I wasn't terribly passionate about it, and I knew that I wanted to do something with my life that I was passionate about. Shortly after arriving in L.A., I had joined some of the Australian communities. I figured it would be good to meet some fellow Aussies and as I was navigating my new home, I could learn from others who had been there longer, as I knew that I was sure to have a lot of questions.

At the time, the Australian communities in L.A. held a lot of social events. Unfortunately, over the years they have diminished, but I met some of my closest friends and business colleagues at those events over the years. As an Aussie fresh off the boat, so to speak, these events were invaluable to me. If I was ever feeling a bit homesick or overwhelmed and I went to an event that was surrounded by Aussies, I would automatically feel a sense of belonging – a sense of being home.

At one of the events, I met someone who worked at an Australian Government department in L.A. They asked me what I did, and when I told them they said I could probably offer a unique perspective given my background and experience. They explained they had an issue, had sought legal advice from three different firms and had obtained three completely different answers, so they were at a loss as to what to do. They asked if I might be interested in taking a look. I was intrigued, and of course said I would be happy to, quickly handing over my new business card. The next day there was an email waiting for me with more details of the issue.

In undertaking my review over the months that followed, I actually discovered that the issue presented to me was something that many companies were probably also faced with, albeit without realizing. I also subsequently discovered there was a huge gap in the legal market because (a) at the time, no one seemed to be talking about cross-border legal issues; (b) I couldn't find any other attorney who was doing this type of work; and (c) I quickly discovered there were a lot of people advising on one side of the issue without considering or understanding the legal landscape from a cross-border perspective.

What a lot of companies did not appreciate is the extent of legal issues that can arise when companies are operating across multiple jurisdictions. I realized those same companies would typically obtain legal advice from a firm in a local market, and then get advice from another firm in another local market, and the advice may end up incorrect or with gaps because the cross-border elements had not been considered. In some situations, there may be conflicting law or overlapping law that needed to be considered and addressed as well.

What I have found is that generally only a lawyer that is qualified in, or really understands the cross-border, international context gets this. I advised the firm on that issue, and then another and another. The initial client referred me to others having similar issues, and so my network and practice continued to grow. Eventually I ended up giving up U.S. litigation all together, although I do still litigate a small number of cases today where they involve multi-national companies and/or cross-border issues.

The main focus areas of my practice now though are market entry, advising companies with international expansion, and assisting companies to manage their business and people on a global scale. It has been an incredible journey that has presented me with opportunities that I would never have imagined had I not moved to the U.S. I have been to cities right across the U.S. for work, including San Francisco, Dallas, San Diego, New York, Hershey, Austin, Seattle and many more, as well as the U.K., Ireland, Canada, and Brazil. You might say that during my time in the U.S., I really have learnt how to turn those lemons into margaritas! A skill that has definitely served me well, as further, arguably more difficult events in my life have transpired since then.

For anyone considering an international career move in the future, I'd say don't waste time considering it – jump in headfirst! Whether you end up loving the job and establishing a life in another country or not, is not really important. The main thing is the experience of living life in another country, learning different cultures from other people with different experiences to you, which is invaluable and something that can never be experienced other than through living it. I also really believe that people who have lived an expat life generally make the best employees because they bring unique experiences and perspectives to the workplace. They are often able to think out issues and problem solve in different ways because they have experienced differences in cultures and that directly impacts the workplace environment. It also changes you. Forever you will be an expat with life experiences, colleagues, and friends in different parts of the world, and that is really special. So, my advice is that if you are an employee that is ever faced with the decision to work in another country – take the leap! If you are a company that is considering global expansion, do it today. But plan, get advice and don't cut corners. And if you are an employer who comes across a job applicant who has overseas experience, hire them!

My practice continued to go from strength to strength, and it has expanded over time as my skills and experience have also grown and developed as well. I now assist companies from all over the world and am very proud to be able to say that I have assisted over 400 companies with their international operations.

Being Found

In January 2015, I attended the Australia Day Gala in San Francisco. The event was something I attended every year, as some of my clients typically went and it was also a great way to connect with potential new clients and other Aussies in the U.S. as well. That year I went with my friend Sarah, who lives in San Francisco. We sat at a table with a number of people from Telstra and Dave (now my husband) was also seated at the table. Now, these types of events are really work for me, so while I always have a good time, my main priority is to meet people, make new connections and ensure that my clients enjoy themselves.

As such, when Dave approached me, although I was nice, I did make it clear that I was there for work, not to meet somebody that night. I was also happy and I really had not dated anyone seriously after my last horrifying relationship. I felt that it wasn't fair to commit to someone until I had healed after my last experience. I also wanted to be 100 percent sure that nightmare was in fact completely over. I certainly didn't want to be the cause of anyone getting hurt or harassed because of me. So, on that night I politely made it clear I wasn't interested.

However, Dave was persistent, and he was really very sweet. I gave in and ended up spending some of the night talking to him. We even went for drinks afterwards with some other friends who were at the Gala. At the end of the night, Dave said that he would like to come and see me in L.A, so I gave him my number, but really had no expectations. I honestly didn't expect to hear from him again. However, a day or so later, Dave did call, and to my surprise, told me that he had booked a ticket to L.A. for the following weekend. He told me he was going to arrive on Friday afternoon and asked if I might be able to collect him from the airport.

I was a bit shell shocked after my past experiences, but I decided I should give Dave a chance and so I agreed. Despite my initial reservations, in the end the weekend went well, and pretty quickly,

Dave and I were inseparable. We really hit it off and we had a shared experience in that we were both Aussies living in the U.S. as expats, working for large corporations. We ended up spending almost every weekend together, with me going up to San Francisco or Dave coming down to L.A. Four months later, Dave asked me to go to Turkey with him, as he was going to meet some of his friends from Australia there and they were going sailing for a week. I had never been to Turkey, and I was having such a good time with Dave getting to know him that I immediately said yes.

Before heading to Turkey, we went to Australia together and Dave met my family, as he attended my cousin's wedding with me. My brother Josh had joked that Dave would probably propose in Turkey, which I laughed off, thinking it would never happen. Little did I know that Dave had in fact already bought a promise ring to propose with. He had planned a ring he could use to propose with but would later let me choose what ring I wanted. So, on May 28, on the top of Saint Nicholas Island in Turkey, Dave did indeed propose to me. And, without hesitation, instantly I said, "Yes!".

No marriage is perfect. It takes work. At times it is wonderful. At times it is challenging. I have my quirks and annoying habits, just as Dave does. However, finding Dave, after everything I had been through, felt like such a blessing and had I not ended up in L.A., I would probably never have ended up married to Dave. It is so hard to understand why we go through challenges in life sometimes, but the important thing is not to forget, but rather to try to use the experiences to move forward in your life in some positive way. I have tried to live my life like this and to be an example for others. I haven't always gotten it right. I have made plenty of mistakes along this journey that we call life, and that's okay. In my view though, the most important thing is to learn a lesson, get back up, keep moving forward and use the experience to change our lives for the better, and hopefully, also make positive changes for others in the process too.

When Trying for Milk You Drink a Lot of Margaritas

Dave and I were older when we met, and we were both on the same page about wanting to start a family right away. I got pregnant fairly quickly and we were really excited. That excitement was short-lived, as I lost the baby just as quickly. The second time we were pregnant, everything seemed to be progressing well. Due to the nature of my practice, I travel a lot for work, and I was almost four months pregnant when I had to go back to Australia. It was going to be a pretty grueling trip with events and meetings in five states over three weeks. I was also in the middle of a large Federal Court post-employment restraint case that was set for hearing in Brisbane during those three weeks as well, so it was going to be a non-stop trip.

Brisbane was my first destination because of the trial. Shortly after I arrived, I noticed some bleeding. I rushed to a hospital and underwent some testing, after which the hospital told me the baby was fine, but said I would need to continue monitoring with an OBGYN. The doctors also said I would need to continue scans every few days until I was able to return home and see my own doctor in L.A. I asked the hospital doctor whether I was at risk, with the amount of travel that I had to complete in a short period of time, but she assured me there was no evidence that flying is detrimental to a baby in utero, so I continued on.

I did, however, make sure I saw a doctor in each city I visited and I stuck to the recommended schedule of a new scan every two to three days to ensure the baby was still doing okay. I also had regular blood tests throughout the trip to check that my HSGC levels remained in the normal range, based on my baby's gestational age. Everything seemed normal. The baby had a strong heartbeat and I continued with the roadshow without further incident. That was, at least until my final weekend in Melbourne.

When I am back in Australia for work, I typically try to spend my weekends in Melbourne so that I can be with my family and catch up with friends. There is never a trip home without at least making time to see my mother, my brothers and my good friends Sharon, Georg, James, and Karl. On this trip though, I had arranged to catch up with a lot of friends I hadn't seen for some time. We were all meeting at a restaurant at the St. Kilda Sea Baths and I was excited to see everyone. I arrived about an hour earlier, as I planned to first take a walk with a coffee, along the beach.

I had just ordered the coffee when I suddenly felt wet. I went to the bathroom and discovered a LOT of blood. I panicked! I was quite sure I had lost the baby this time. I called my mother and she asked me whether I thought I could drive. I was shaken, but we agreed it would be quicker for her to meet me at the hospital rather than come all the way to St. Kilda to collect me first.

When I arrived and told them what had happened, they rushed me straight in for a scan. My mother arrived just as I had been prepped. We were both so relieved when the doctor told us that the baby appeared to be fine. She could not see any signs of distress and the baby's heartbeat remained strong. I told the doctor about what had happened during the last few weeks, and she explained to me that some women just experience some bleeding throughout their pregnancy, for no particular reason. She thought it probably wasn't anything to worry about. I told the doctor I was due to fly home to L.A. the next morning and she said I should arrange to see my doctor as soon as I arrived back in L.A., but as everything appeared to be okay, I could go home.

I called my doctor's office in L.A. to book an appointment a few hours after my flight was scheduled to arrive back into LAX. I didn't sleep well that night though, as I was worried about the baby and concerned about how much bleeding had occurred earlier that day. I was also really sad to be leaving my family, especially mum, as I really wanted her with me in light of stress of the pregnancy difficulties I was experiencing. The next morning, I flew home with a heavy heart. I was restless on the flight back and felt a bit unwell. When I arrived in L.A. I went straight from the airport to see my doctor. I told the doctor what had been going on, and the first thing she said to me was, "I don't understand why no one gave you a steroid injection. They should have done that. It helps in these circumstances, just in case."

I will never forget lying down on that table for the scan only to hear nothing. Silence. There was no heartbeat. My baby had passed away. All I could hear was the sound of my own screams and tears, although they appeared to be coming from someone else outside of my body. The doctor hugged me and Dave and I cried. I didn't understand what had gone wrong, but I knew without a doubt that my baby had passed away while I was mid-air, on my way back to LA. I just knew it in my heart. Of course, at the time I also blamed myself and thought I should not have flown such a long way under the circumstances, but whether it would have made a difference or not, I will never know.

Because my baby was about five months along, it meant I had to have surgery. The doctor scheduled the procedure a few days later. I still recall that day vividly, because up until that point at least, it was the hardest day of my life. I should have been in that hospital to have my baby a few months later, not to be there then to say goodbye. I cried my heart out.

Something happened that day though, that I will never forget. As my doctor and the anesthesiologist wheeled me into the operating theatre, they held each of my hands and said a little prayer with me. They both had tears in their eyes.

"I'm so sorry sweetheart," the lovely anesthesiologist said. "Now let me take that pain away for you, for just a little while. Close your eyes and rest now."

And that is what I did, with tears running down my cheeks and the two doctors holding my hands. I will never forget that act of human kindness. It was beautiful and so very much appreciated.

My Eligh

I had asked the doctor to perform an autopsy on my baby that day. I had to know whether there was something wrong with my baby or if it was me. I felt it was important information. I needed to know if I was ever going to be able to have a child of my own. I also wanted to know whether our baby was a boy or a girl. The doctor tried to talk me out of it, but I felt these were important things for me to know. I felt it would help with my healing as well. My baby had been a little boy.

Eligh was one of the boys' names that was on our baby list and the one that both Dave and I could actually agree on. So, although we did not officially name the baby, he will always be Eligh to me. The doctor also told me that the baby had not had any medical issues to explain why he had passed away. There was nothing wrong with Eligh. What the doctor discovered though, is that the baby had not been getting sufficient food from my body and essentially, he had starved. All I could think was, "Oh my God! I killed my baby".

For weeks afterwards, I hated myself. I hated this body of mine that could not feed my baby. I spent the next few weeks in bed, but I worked right through. My body and mind felt exhausted, and everything felt numb. Those weeks went by in a blur; it was as if I was on autopilot. I couldn't understand how the world around me continued on, as if nothing was different, when everything in my world had changed. I was angry and I was quite sure I was never going to be the same again.

At the time, of course, my boss told me to take whatever time off work I needed, and I was probably also asked if any client work needed to be managed in my absence. I can't recall the exact details of the few emails I exchanged with my boss, but I know I didn't take more than a day or two off. I told my boss I would be okay. I would manage. As the only qualified Australian lawyer in the firm at the time, there wasn't anyone else to assist with my work and I suppose that is probably why no alternatives were presented to me. So, I just pushed through and carried on – but I now question whether that was the right approach.

Honestly, I should not have said I would be okay. I should not have just tried to push through without regard to the needs of my body or mind. I should have taken more time to rest and recover both physically and mentally. Equally, there were probably things the firm could have done better to manage the situation as well. I don't say this to be critical. It is simply the reality because most organizations have significant room to improve in this area of employee relations. Legally though, this type of situation is an incredibly difficult one to manage, because what an employer really should say in that type of scenario is: "We don't think that it is in your best interest to work right now. We don't want you to have to worry about work. We want you to focus on your recovery." However, taking action like that is fraught with risk, because doing so carries a degree of discrimination.

In my view, a much better approach would be to provide the employee with support, encourage them to take time off, and offer them some alternative options that might be suitable in the circumstances. For example, in my case, looking back now, what would have assisted me at the time would have been someone assigned to simply manage the client emails that were coming in during that time. While it was likely inevitable that I would have had to continue doing some work regardless, reducing the contact I had to have with people during that time would have provided me with additional time and space to focus on my own wellness. I also would have been much more likely to take some time away from work if some options had been presented to me.

The problem is that in times of personal tragedy or illness, when we ask someone if they are okay, the natural reaction that most of us will provide is, "I'm fine" or "I'll be okay", when in reality that response is far from the truth. By changing the narrative slightly, and instead making a statement such as, "I can't imagine what you must be going through right now. Please know that we are here to support you in any way that we can. We want to encourage you to take the time you need without having to worry about work, so here are some suggestions for how we can assist you during this time."

This places the employee in a situation where they are empowered to make decisions about what they need, but it also enables them to do so in a way that feels much more comfortable, supported and inclusive, because it demonstrates that the organization has taken the time to think through the situation and work out ways to assist. That type of small difference in approach can make a significant difference to an employee who is experiencing things such as grief, serious illness or loss.

Losing a baby is something that is tragically experienced by so many people each year. It is estimated that one in four pregnancies end in a loss. Yet, despite these statistics being so high, it is amazing that it still remains a topic that is so rarely discussed in public forums, and even less so in the workplace context. So why is it that we still live in societies where these types of issues are considered to be private, and that we should keep them to ourselves, yet we ask people to come to work and be their whole authentic selves?

Throughout my years of practice as a lawyer, I have reviewed a LOT of workplace policies. I am always astonished when I see policies that include statements such as, "We want our employees to be authentic" or "We have a culture here where employees can bring their whole selves to work" because in my experience most employers do not actually want this at all. What they really want is for their employees to come to work and leave their problems at home. Sure, employers are happy to hear that Joe is a new father and Mary is a new mother, but they generally don't want to hear the difficulties that come along with those roles, and when it comes to divorce, breakups and health issues, most companies generally want to know about it even less.

What they want is for their employees to be able to leave their personal problems at the door, enter the workplace and perform their jobs without regard to the impact of their personal lives. Most employers just don't want their employees to bring their personal issues to work. You might be thinking that sounds very cynical, but as an employment lawyer, I see this scenario played out frequently. Although I have seen statements like this included in policies hundreds of times, I must admit I am still unsure exactly what the organizations actually mean by those statements. I also do not understand what companies including a statement like this are hoping it will achieve.

One thing that I do know, is that words have little meaning without action, and employees cannot be fooled. An organization cannot have policies that state all the right things and then have practices and a culture that foster a lack of support for their employees, or worse, bullying, harassment and discrimination. In fact, for these types of companies, it would be better to say nothing in their policies at all.

Loss and grief are very real things, and we know that these things impact everyone differently. Therefore the needs of employees when they are experiencing a tragedy or trauma in their lives will differ. That is just reality, and I do appreciate that this can make it challenging to implement policies and benefits plans that will work for every employee in every situation. However, we can apply that type of logic to almost every situation, so if we use that as an excuse to do nothing, then nothing would ever get done and there would be no progress for the better.

We can never make every person happy. The point is that there are improvements that every single company and every single manager can make to better support employees at work. Implementing a policy or practice that assists women to return to the workplace, to remain in the workplace, or to succeed in the workplace is well worth the effort for many reasons, as I will discuss in more detail throughout this book.

Our Fertility Journey

When I think back to the days and weeks following the loss of my baby, I feel sadness and disappointment, but not just because of the loss of my baby. Of course, I will always feel sadness for the child that I lost and wonder what my little boy would have looked like and the person he would have become; I also feel disappointed in myself. Putting aside the fact that I should have taken the time that I needed to rest and heal from the experience that I was going through, I also failed other women around me. You see, as a woman in a leadership position, I believe that I have an obligation to set positive examples for other women to follow, and I am here to say that I did a poor job of it during that time. It is actually one of the reasons why I was led to start presenting on the topic of women's health issues and the workplace, and ultimately write this book to share my experiences with you.

I want to tell you that I was wrong. In the days, weeks and months that followed the loss of my baby – the surgeries, procedures, and fertility treatments – I set an example for others. I didn't stop pushing myself. I just kept working and pushed myself through. I tried to be 'tough'. I didn't want to let anyone down. I didn't want anyone to think of me as weak, incapable, or unreliable. I didn't want to be a failure. And you know what? Not one person told me not to do it. Not one person told me to stop. To focus on me. To lean into my loss. No one insisted I focus on dealing with my grief and not to worry about the rest of the world around me for just a little while.

And you see, I have now realized that what I was actually doing was not effectively dealing with my loss or grief at all, and I was inadvertently setting an expectation for myself, and worse, a bad example for others. I am now here to tell you that what I did is definitely NOT the example to follow! The problem is that it provided validation for people to think that if I could do it, then others should be able to do it as well. Right? And, if they couldn't, then does that make them weak, incapable, unreliable? The answer is, no – definitely not! My actions fed into the narrative though, that to be successful, to be a 'good' employee, you cannot show weakness. You simply must show up and continue on, no matter how broken you might be on the inside, both physically and mentally.

About a week or so after the procedure, I saw my doctor for a post-op examination, and I am not ashamed to tell you that I cried throughout the entire appointment. Hormone levels rapidly change after a miscarriage and it typically takes at least a few weeks, if not longer, for a woman's hormones to level out again after pregnancy. Mood swings and tears are normal, even without factoring in the profound grief that follows the loss of a baby.

Ultimately though, I wasn't dealing with my loss effectively because I wasn't allowing myself any time at all to do so. I was so worried about letting others down, not appearing weak or unreliable to my firm, keeping my clients happy and meeting their needs, that I was completely neglecting my own. Sure, people checked in with me from time to time during that period to see if I was okay, but what was I going to say? "No, actually I am not. I can't sleep. I can't stop crying. I just want my baby!"

The other thing I realized about appearing 'strong', is that others naturally start assuming you must be fine too. While you may be dying inside – to the outside world the expectations remain the same and the effect is that the workplace stresses that, under normal circumstances may have been tolerable, all of a sudden start to chip away – until one day that hard exterior just cracks! And when it cracks, boy, is there going to be a big explosion!

We need to stop 'checking in' to see if people are 'okay' and start having meaningful interactions with our employees when they experience loss, grief, and heartache. We need to stop avoiding difficult and uncomfortable conversions and start offering real, tangible options, resources, and support to employees, through things like workplace flexibility and the ability to take time away from work to deal with grief – without fear of repercussions or job loss. We should be making women who are experiencing fertility issues, child loss, menopause and other women's health issues feel comfortable and confident enough to raise their hands when they need their employer's help, instead of buying into the narrative that women who need support or assistance are weak or unreliable. Yet, disappointingly, there are so few examples that I have seen in workplaces that are really doing this effectively.

My doctor could see that I was suffering and so she asked me if I was ready to talk about the next steps. She said she thought it might be what I needed, to work out a plan to move forward, to try again. I agreed it might be best, and she said she often referred high risk patients to Dr. Carrie Wambach. Dr. Wambach is an IVF doctor with fantastic experience in assisting couples with reproductive issues to have successful pregnancies. So, off I went to see Dr. Wambach a few days later.

I instantly loved her. She was kind and supportive and immediately made me feel at ease because she is quite open about her own experiences in having her family. When you are going through the pain of losing a child, and you are experiencing difficulties having children, this is the type of support and understanding that really helps. It is also one of the reasons why I believe I have been so successful in my practice as a lawyer, because I am able to relate to my clients and their experiences. I not only advise companies on their market-entry journeys, but I can speak from personal experience about my own journey from Australia to the U.S., to the U.K. and back to the U.S. again.

I understand and empathize with my clients' challenges because I too have lived them, and I celebrate their successes, as I know the hard work and commitment that is involved in breaking into, and ultimately finding, success in a new market. People are drawn to human connection and a deep understanding and my view on business is that to really be successful, you need to find that type of connection with your clients, that thing that makes you unique. In other words, what is your story and how can you use it to relate to others? When you find a way to connect with your clients, you can create lasting relationships. They become friends, not just clients, and ultimately that makes the difference between a short-term transaction and a lasting relationship.

It is also really important to never take any client for granted, and in fact one of my aims to is make sure that every single one of them feels as if they are my one and only client. Each one is as important to me as the next. I am always really thankful when clients will say things to me like, "I may only contact you every six months or so, but thank you for always answering my emails me so promptly every time." That makes me feel as if I am making a difference in the work I do, and honestly, I think that is something that we should all be striving for in one way or another in life.

Dr. Wambach ran many tests on me over the next few weeks. She wanted to be thorough and eliminate absolutely every possible issue that could explain why I had lost my baby, and why I was having problems carrying a pregnancy to term. We knew at that stage that I had been born with a blood condition called Von Willebrand's Disease, but that disease is typically not something that impacts fertility. The body makes higher amounts of Von Willebrand and other clotting factors during pregnancy to prevent bleeding, so Dr. Wambach didn't believe that was causing the problem. I also have endometriosis but again, that didn't appear to be the cause of the issue because I was getting pregnant, although of course we will never really know for sure.

At the end of the testing, I met with Dr. Wambach in her office, and she was perplexed. She knew there had to be some explanation for the problems I was experiencing, but she couldn't find anything wrong with me despite the extensive testing. I remember watching her that day. She was so intently focused and was clearly searching through her head, trying to think about what it could possibly be. After some time, deep in thought, she suddenly looked up and said, "There is one test that I didn't run on you. Because you have Von Willebrand's, it would be extremely unlikely that you could have a clotting condition. However, I have eliminated everything else that I can possibly think of, so for the sake of completeness, let's run that test." I was feeling rather deflated and exhausted at this point and I was starting to think that maybe we would never be able to have children but, nonetheless, away I went for more blood tests.

I went home and lay on the sofa that afternoon. I continued to respond to work emails that were urgent, but I didn't have the energy to sit at a desk that day. I felt completely defeated and I was anxious while awaiting the blood test results because I had no idea where we were going to go from here. Sometime late in the afternoon, I received a call from Dr. Wambach. Sure enough, the test came back to show that I had a clotting Factor-5 deficiency. So, I had a bleeding disorder and a clotting disorder that was likely causing an issue. We now had some possible answers, as well as some options.

Unfortunately, the two conditions together posed an additional problem. It meant that it was going to be very difficult to treat, because anything that the hematologist could provide me for one condition would be problematic for the other. I am thankful that my doctors were so willing to work together to try to assist me and they were able to formulate a combined plan for my care. This is something I am incredibly grateful for, because I know it doesn't often happen. In the end, Dr Wambach and my hematologist, Dr Sadeghi, both agreed I would undertake a round of IVF with an intense dose of blood thinning injections each day. As they said, I was going to be in for a wild ride!

There are many different types and methods of IVF, including a natural cycle, mild stimulation, and in vitro maturation, and these can vary in both the process, requirements, and duration. For me, my IVF process involved a three-week period, during which I was injecting myself daily for about ten to twelve days, and attending appointments about every second day for scans and blood tests, as well as additional appointments with my hematologist. With the blood thinning injections, which were the size and thickness of an injection that you might expect some large animal to receive, not a human, I was injecting myself eight times a day.

I was extremely sick from all of the hormones and my stomach was covered in bruises. I spent weeks in bed throwing up, my head throbbing with pain. My body felt bloated, and I was all over the place emotionally with the surge of hormones that were entering my body each day. I felt wretched, but I pushed through. There was no other option.

When you are sick as a dog, three weeks is a very long time, but somehow I found the will to carry on. I would be lying though if I said I didn't think about giving up. There were a few close calls during those difficult days, when I told Dave I just couldn't keep going and I actually meant it. Dave was very supportive and told me that if I didn't want to do it, then I didn't have to. He said it was entirely my decision, which I really appreciated, but ultimately, I knew our insurance only covered three rounds of IVF and if I gave up halfway through a cycle, then I would be ruining one of our crucial chances to have a family, so I continued on and made it through. I was so thankful when the day of the retrieval surgery finally arrived. It felt like a huge relief, as I knew there would be no more injections and I could finally let my body start to recover.

There is typically some pain and discomfort after egg retrieval surgery, although it does vary from one person to the next. As someone who has lived my life with varying degrees of pain associated with my endometriosis, the pain following the retrieval procedure was nothing particularly out of the ordinary for me. It was just another Monday. But one of the worst parts of the IVF process is the period of waiting post-retrieval. Each day you wait for a call from the doctor to give you the status update – how many eggs were retrieved? What were they graded? How many resulted in viable embryos? How many survived day one, day three and beyond; through to blastocyst stage, on about day five or six? There were so many questions to be answered.

Three days after fertilization, a normally developing embryo will contain about six to ten cells. By the fifth or sixth day, the fertilized egg is known as a blastocyst – a rapidly dividing ball of cells. The inner group of cells will become the embryo. The outer group will become the cells that nourish and protect it. The blastocyst will ultimately hatch from the protective 'shell', which has surrounded the embryo through its early development. This is called the zona pellucida. It is this mass of hatched cells which, once free from its shell, will implant into the lining of the womb and form a pregnancy. Blastocyst is what you want to aim for, and good quality eggs with gradings A or B have the highest chance of making it through to this stage – although, I do have friends who have only ended up with C grade eggs and have still had children. Anything can happen in IVF!

The news on day one, after the egg retrieval surgery, was that we had a lot of high-quality grade A and B eggs. I can't actually recall how many we ended up with, but it was at least twelve. By blastocyst stage on day five and six, we had about six female and three male embryos. We decided to have preimplantation genetic testing performed on our embryos because we were fortunate to have such a high number. The testing determines whether the embryos are genetically normal and healthy, and as the majority of pregnancy losses that occur in the first trimester are due to embryo aneuploidy, this type of testing provides an additional layer of protection, as it enables you to select the strongest, most viable embryos for implantation.

The downside to conducting genetic testing at this stage though, is that there is some risk that the embryo can be destroyed as a result of the testing and there are typically additional costs associated with the testing, which may not be covered by insurance plans that provide for IVF treatments. For us though, we decided that we did not want to leave anything to chance, and we felt it was better to know which embryos would provide us with the best chance of having a child. After the testing, we ended up with three female and one male embryo and we decided to implant two – one male and one female. I started the meds in preparation for the transfer and the date was set. We were on our way to the final stage, or at least I hoped we were.

The day of transfer was exciting. I felt full of hope and had a confidence that I had not felt for a long time. The transfer was quick and painless, and Dave was there watching through a microscope, as the little embryos were selected, placed into the catheter and away they went, with us both saying a little prayer for their journey. I was told to go home and relax as much as possible. I asked whether I should put my legs in the air or lie upside down, or with my backside raised like I had seen in so many movies, but the doctor just laughed and told me that none of those things were necessary, staying calm and relaxed with no physical exertion was key.

The transfer was done on a Thursday, so we decided to go away to Palm Springs for the weekend, as it is one of our favorite semi-local getaway destinations and there is not a lot to do there but rest, read a book and look at the desert scenery. We invited some friends and rented a large house together. It was a lovely few days of relaxing, eating, drinking – (sans alcohol for me!) – good conversation and lots of laughter. It was exactly what I needed, and I felt so sure that I was now pregnant with our two little seeds and that I was going to be a mother of boy and girl twins.

I spent much of the weekend fantasizing about what they were going to look like, what their names would be, what their rooms would look like and all of the wonderful things that we would do together as a family. I could not wait! It came as a complete shock to my system when I returned to Los Angeles a few days later to attend my first appointment after the transfer, only to be told that the HSCG levels in my blood indicated that the transfer probably had not been successful. Dr. Wambach told me not to lose hope just yet. She told me to come back the following day for another test to see whether the levels had risen, but I already knew in my heart what it meant, and this was confirmed the next day when the blood test showed with no uncertainty that the HSCG levels had dropped even further. Our little seeds had not made it. I was not pregnant! Once again, my body had failed us, and I was sad. I was devastated and totally gutted with utter disappointment.

I remember the day very clearly, just like it was yesterday. Dave's Aunt and Uncle were in L.A. on vacation at the time and they were staying with us for a few days. I had just received the dreaded phone call to confirm the news that I already knew in my heart, and I was lying on the sofa in a fetal position, wailing my heart out like an animal screaming in pain. I was in agony. I had a pain in my chest that felt exactly as if my heart had exploded right down the middle, broken into two pieces. Dave's Aunt walked in to find me like this, and she didn't know what to say. What could anyone say? There was nothing that was going to make me feel better. I just needed to cry.

Thinking back to that day now, I almost feel as though I am looking at myself from the corner of the room and I feel like crying as I write this. It is still raw and extremely painful. I wasn't crying just for the loss of those two little embryos. I was crying for all of the months and months of heartache and disappointment that we had experienced. I was crying for all of the tests, scans, doctors' appointments, hospital visits, surgeries, injections, hormones, poking, prodding, loss of dignity, ups, downs and babies that I had lost. I was crying because I think that I knew then that my body was broken. It wasn't capable of carrying a baby and I didn't know why. I didn't understand what I had done to deserve such a fate. I felt broken in so many ways and I also felt like I was letting Dave down too. Becoming a parent was after all not just my dream, but something that he wanted badly as well. I felt as though I had disappointed him and that it wasn't fair to ask him to stay with me. After all, he had bought broken goods and so I told him that he didn't have to stay, that I would understand if he wanted to leave me because I couldn't give him what he deserved.

All of these things that I was thinking and feeling were reasonable and unreasonable, rational and irrational, and although it was fair enough to feel this way, I was being completely unfair to myself. It was a lot to cope with all at once. Of course, Dave told me not to think that way at all, that I was not a disappointment and that he had not married me for my ability to have children. He told me that he loved me regardless of whether we were able to have a family or not and that we would just have to find another way.

I love him for that, because not every person would have that same attitude. I know couples who have not survived this type of news, with one person ultimately deciding to walk away. I do not judge those people at all. Everyone has to make whatever decisions they feel are right for their own lives, but I will always be grateful to Dave that he never even considered walking away. He was with me, supporting me every step of the way. The doctor called that evening to see how I was doing after hearing in my voice how devastated I was.

"I really think we need to consider other options now," he said. "I don't think your body, or your heart can take any more. I think you should consider surrogacy."

Dave immediately said, "Let's do it!" without a moment's hesitation. Dave, I love you for that and so much more.

IVF is expensive, but surrogacy is something on another level. Expensive is an understatement. It is a huge financial commitment. Much like buying a house, except an even more significant investment because (a) it is an investment in family and your future; and (b) it is an investment that carries a high risk of getting no return. Regardless, we didn't care. We were one-hundred percent aligned in our view that we absolutely had to find a way to make it work. We are fortunate that Dave's parents agreed to help us with the cost, so it was one less thing we needed to worry about, and this actually made starting the process fairly quick and painless for us. We were also extremely fortunate to have such an amazing doctor in Dr. Wambach because she went above and beyond in her attempts to help us. Dr. Wambach knew how much we were grieving and how much I had been through in such a short period of time. She wanted us to succeed because she had been there herself. She knew exactly what this kind of heartache felt like and that makes her one special doctor.

There were also other issues at play. My body had not responded well to the drugs, and I am almost positive that the combination of the IVF process with the stress I was under is what led to the additional problems I ended up facing. It was one issue after another. Fibroids, polyps, cysts, painful endometriosis. What I ultimately really needed was to have a hysterectomy, but that just wasn't an option at that time. I went through one surgery after the next and I had a number of days when I would awaken only to find I couldn't stand up. It was a new symptom for me and not something I had experienced before, as a result of my endometriosis. I get bad back pain from the endometriosis to this day, but during that period it was different. There were days when I literally could not stand up straight. The pain was unbearable.

At one point during this period, my gynecologist had scheduled me for more surgery in about seven days and while waiting for the surgery I ended up being rushed to the ER in excruciating pain. My doctor ended up operating that same day. One of the benefits of the U.S. healthcare system, (I am well aware that there are many problems with U.S. healthcare, but this is definitely a real positive!) is that if you go to the ER of the medical group that your doctor is affiliated with, your doctor can come in and perform the surgery then and there. You don't get assigned to a doctor you don't know.

I was dealing with my own physical health issues, broken-hearted and struggling to find the will to keep moving forward with our family plan, all while trying to manage a busy legal practice and keep my head above water. There was little time to stop, little time to enjoy being newlyweds, and zero time for self-care. It was not a great situation, but I know that it is typical of what so many women who are experiencing fertility issues are going through every day. My fertility journey is unfortunately not unique. One in eight women are believed to experience fertility issues globally. And this is exactly why understanding this statistic and the impact that fertility issues can have on a woman and her career is so crucial to the issue of gender equality. If we are ever going to move ahead towards closing the gap, then we simply must start thinking about women and the workplace in a different way. It is not simply a nice thing to do, it is an absolutely essential discussion.

Our Surrogacy Journey

Surrogacy is a complex issue. Over the years since my daughters were born, I have spoken publicly about this topic a number of times. I have advised many clients on issues surrounding surrogacy employee benefit plans and I am now on the Board of Surrogacy Australia. I have learnt a lot through research, my own experience, and the work that I now do to advocate for change in this area. I have also learnt just how many legal challenges and strong differences of opinion exist when it comes to this topic, and I have found it fascinating to discover that it seems to be one of those things where people generally have very strong opinions on whether it is right or wrong.

For some reason, there is a group of opponents of surrogacy who have strong beliefs about why they consider it unnatural, against God's will or just generally wrong. I can tell you because I have spoken to a number of media publications on the issue of surrogacy over the years and every single time there are trolls who write horrible and offensive comments on the story. I have heard everything from, "If God meant for you to have children, then you would have been able to have one", to "You're an evil person for buying your children and I hope that you die!". Believe me, there are some really horrible people out there who will write terrible things from behind the safety of their computer screen.

There have also been others who have politely engaged in discussion with me about their views and have respectfully listened to mine. Sometimes I am able to convince them as to why it is not something to be feared and is something that is needed in certain circumstances, and other times I am not and that's okay. In life we are never going to have the same views, values, and beliefs as everyone in the entire world. I wouldn't want to live in a world like that. What a boring place that would be and when we don't have people to continually challenge us and our ideas and beliefs. Then we would have no motivation to strive, to seek improvement, and to think of ways to continue to make positive changes.

Whenever you decide to become an advocate for change, you are always going to come up against opposition. There are a few reasons for this. Firstly, as I just mentioned, there is never going to be any issue that one-hundred percent of the world's population see eye-to-eye on, but when you break it down further, there are reasons for that. Most people do not like change. Humans are creatures of habit. It is the reason why we end up with cultures and traditions that can last hundreds and even thousands of years. We like security and safety and those things that are known to us are comfortable and therefore we typically develop similar views and proceed in similar patterns and ways of life as our parents, grandparents, and theirs before them.

Independently, culture also plays a significant role in many of the women's health issues that I talk about throughout the book. I touch on the issue of culture in more detail in Chapter 6, but it should not be underestimated in discussions around these types of topics. As an expat myself, having lived in three countries, Australia, the U.S., and the U.K., I have seen this first-hand. For example, in the U.S., surrogacy is so widely utilized, that no one really bats an eyelid when it is mentioned. It is certainly not something that is limited to celebrities either. In my own circle of friends, we know three separate couples who have all undertaken surrogacy to have their children. The states set surrogacy laws in the U.S. and the legal systems in every state except Nebraska, Louisiana, and Michigan are set up to effectively handle both commercial and altruistic gestational, and traditional surrogacy cases. Arizona and Indiana are also problematic states, because while surrogacy is practiced and courts issue parentage orders, surrogacy contracts are void and unenforceable by statute.

In the U.K. the situation is somewhat different. Surrogacy is legal in the U.K., but if you make a surrogacy agreement, it cannot be enforced by the law. The surrogate will be the child's legal parent at birth. If the surrogate is married or in a civil partnership, their spouse or civil partner will be the child's second parent at birth, unless they did not give their permission. Legal parenthood can be transferred by parental order or adoption after the child is born and if there is disagreement about who the child's legal parents should be, the courts will make a decision about parentage based on the best interests of the child.

In New Zealand it is similar to Australia, the laws are complex, and children born via surrogacy can spend at least their first months after birth in a legal limbo without a legal parent at law. Current law states that egg or sperm donors are not legal parents. This leaves four potential legal parents: the surrogate, her partner and the intended parent or parents. Thankfully, a Law Commission review[6] has been announced in 2021, which proposes significant reform to surrogacy laws in New Zealand.

Australia has a complex legal system when it comes to surrogacy, which is why we have been so strongly advocating for change at Surrogacy Australia. Altruistic surrogacy is legal in most Australian states and territories. Commercial surrogacy, where the surrogate is paid more than the cost of medical and legal expenses, is not legal in most Australian states and territories and in fact commercial surrogacy constitutes a crime in three states. In New South Wales, Queensland and the Australian Capital Territory, it is an offence to enter into a commercial surrogacy arrangement with potential penalties extending to imprisonment for up to one year in the Australian Capital Territory, up to two years imprisonment in New South Wales and up to three years in Queensland.

There have been some positive changes over recent years, as one case or another has come to light, and the topic has risen to the surface of people's minds once again. However, statistically the percentage of Australians who engage in surrogacy each year is so small that it is not generally a topic that is high on any politician's agenda and that is part of the challenge that we face when advocating for change. It is also a challenge when deciding to embark on a surrogacy journey from within Australia because you either have to find a friend or relative to kindly offer you their womb and allow you to take over their body for nine months, or you have to source a stranger to allow you to do this for free (not a particularly easy task for either party when it is a situation that involves so much trust). The only other alternative is to try to navigate a complicated process overseas, while living in Australia and traveling back and forth. It is

---

6. https://www.lawcom.govt.nz/our-projects/review-of-surrogacy

one of the reasons why there is not a higher utilization of surrogacy by Australians. In my view, none of these are great options. However, more on that later.

Of course, when Dr. Wambach suggested surrogacy to us on that day back in 2016, we had no idea about any of this. Sure, we had friends in the U.S. who had undertaken the process, but we hadn't really thought a lot about it other than how great it was that they were able to have a child after such a long struggle with infertility, and one day they were on their own and the next they were with a baby. I never really considered asking many questions about the process, the legal aspect or anything else for that matter because it wasn't something that I ever anticipated needing to know. I certainly did not think at any time in my life, *Wow, surrogacy looks great. It would be an easier option. I wouldn't have to go through a pregnancy and ruin my body*, like I am convinced so many people think about those who undertake a surrogacy journey to have children.

I was fragile straight after the unsuccessful embryo transfer, not just because of that failed process, but also because of everything else that I had already gone through leading up to it. Dr. Wambach believed that I needed to direct my attention straight onto the next thing and she was right. However, what I have since realized is that instead of properly dealing with my loss and grief at that time, I pushed it all to the back of my mind, neatly into the box labelled, 'to open later', while I soldiered on to the next task at hand – the surrogacy process. People always say things like, "I wouldn't change anything because I ended up with you", and while I appreciate the sentiment, I don't think it serves anyone if I don't speak honestly about our experience. There is a lot I learnt along the way and definitely some things that I would do differently, had I known then what I know now.

Whether or not to speak freely on this issue in this book and tell the entire truth of our journey is something I have struggled with for some time. It is not because I want to keep anything deliberately private. After all, I am writing a book about my life here. Right? But it is because I want so desperately for positive change to occur in the area of surrogacy law in Australia that I was concerned about the implications of being so frank, and so publicly. What I don't want is for opponents on this issue to use my story as an example of why surrogacy should remain difficult and commercial surrogacy illegal, because I sincerely believe with all of my heart that that is absolutely the wrong approach.

Dr. Wambach had told us that two of her own children were born via a surrogate and that she had used an agency to assist with sourcing a match and managing the entire process. There are a lot of benefits in using a surrogacy agency because the surrogates undergo a lengthy screening process before they are eligible for matching with a family. There are background checks, counselling sessions and thorough analysis that is conducted with the surrogate and her spouse or partner, if she has one, as they are also obviously impacted by the commitment that is made by being a surrogate for a whole year. The entire screening process can take a year, or even longer in some cases, before the agency will approve the surrogate for matching. Neither my employer nor Dave's provided any type of surrogacy benefits or resources, and this is something now that I advocate for other companies to consider, as a result of our experience. Companies that do offer employee surrogacy benefits can find themselves at a real advantage in the marketplace because to an employee suffering with fertility issues, as well as members of the LGBT+ community, surrogacy benefits can be more valuable than any other benefit or salary that an employer can offer.

We were extremely fortunate that the health insurance benefits that were provided by my firm included three rounds of IVF, which were almost completely covered. The fact that we had access to such great fertility benefits is something I will be forever grateful for. When you are going through an incredibly stressful and emotional time trying to deal with the fact that having children is not possible without intervention, worrying about how you will pay for the medical consultations, testing and treatments that may be required is an additional stress. It is also a huge roadblock that prevents many people from accessing fertility treatments.

Fertility, surrogacy and adoption benefits are excellent drawcards that a lot of progressive companies are now offering their employees as the demand for top talent in certain roles within industries, such as the tech industry, can be fierce. Surrogacy and adoption laws vary significantly across the globe, so it can be challenging for companies to navigate the legal framework that exists within each jurisdiction where they have a presence. However, for those companies that have managed to work through these challenges, they can hold a real advantage in the marketplace. Research conducted by the Reproductive Medicine Associates of New Jersey suggests that sixty-eight percent of adults say that they would switch jobs to gain fertility benefits[7] and a 2018 study conducted by global recruitment experts Korn Ferry[8] found that job applicants no longer care solely about the salary when considering opportunities.

Culture and values currently rank high on the reasons why employees look for new employment. There are many facets to culture and values, but both of these things have a direct correlation to an organization's policies, employee benefits and diversity and inclusion strategies. As most organizations are now placing much more importance on attracting and retaining a diverse workforce, many are now considering how best to support women and minority workers through offering better flexibility and employee benefits, including those focused on family planning, fertility, and childcare support – with some electing to do so through fertility benefit providers such as Carrot[9]. Carrot is a global fertility benefits provider that can assist companies with the implementation and management of these types of employee benefits.

There are a number of other reasons why employer understanding, and support is important, even for companies that do not offer these types of employee benefits. For example, not only is engaging in surrogacy a complex process, but once a person has a child born via surrogate that may not be the end of the legal issues. Just because a person has parental rights in the country where they have undertaken surrogacy, or even within the country where they reside, does not necessarily mean that those rights will be recognized in

7. Infertility in America 2015 Survey and Report by Reproductive Medicine Associates of New Jersey

8. https://www.inc.com/marcel-schwantes/study-top-reason-for-whats-really-driving-employees-to-switch-jobs-in-2018-is-surprising.html

9. https://www.get-carrot.com/

other parts of the world. This has been an issue that has been brought before the European Court of Human Rights for consideration on a number of occasions. The court has had to consider and balance the discretion of countries to implement their own laws with the rights of children born via surrogate, to ensure that they are not denied essential aspects of their identity[10].

For employers, this can become an issue akin to homosexuality and gay marriage. There are similar issues that can arise when employers request that an employee complete an international assignment or short-term work travel to a country that either does not recognize the marriage under its local laws, or where homosexuality is outlawed; which remains the case in approximately seventy countries. It is therefore also an issue that can arise when an employee is asked to undertake international business travel or an international secondment. Employers have a vested interest in ensuring that their employees are well versed in the legal requirements for each relevant country before undertaking a surrogacy or adoption process, otherwise the employee and the employer can find themselves tied up in a legal mess when applying for visas or seeking to send the employee away on international travel.

Dr. Wambach provided us with a list of surrogacy agencies in California and a few interstate options as well. She told us about the one that she had used herself, and so we did not bother looking at any others. If our IVF doctor had used one agency twice, then we figured it must be the best option and that is what we wanted. We didn't want to take any chances. We were also exhausted, so it was far simpler for us to go with a recommendation, rather than spend time going through the various options.

The day that Dr. Wambach provided us with the list we went straight home and called the agency. To my surprise, after telling the women at the agency my name she responded with, "It is great to hear from you. We have been expecting your call." Dr. Wambach had already called the agency and asked them to look after us. She had explained everything that we had gone through, and she did this

---

10. https://papers.ssrn.com/sol3/papers.cfm?abstract_id=3291587

to try and help us because the waitlist for surrogates, especially in locations such as California where demand is high, can be extremely long. It can take more than a year before you reach the top of the list for matching with a surrogate in California.

The agency explained the process in detail for us, they went through all of the costs and also explained that their waitlist for California was currently about eighteen months to two years. I felt immediately deflated until I heard the woman's next words.

"We don't normally do this, but we really feel for you after what Dr. Wambach told us about your story and she asked us to try to help you, so if you are open to considering a surrogate in another state, then I think that we can help you fairly quickly."

That was enough for me! I hadn't actually considered the option of a surrogate in another location. None of the friends who we knew had gone through the process had surrogates outside of California and it just wasn't something I had given any thought to, but I didn't see any reason why it would present any real challenges for us. I was someone who already travelled extensively for work, flights within the U.S. were fairly cheap, and I even thought that it could have some benefits being somewhere else.

What I didn't do though was stop and really think about what it meant and that is where we went wrong. However, we didn't know what we didn't know back then and because of that, I am not sure whether we really could have done anything differently. What I have since learnt is that the location of your surrogate is super important because you are extremely limited in what you can do and how much you can be involved in it. It also means that you have to be prepared to waive some of your decision-making ability if you are not located in the same place as your surrogate, because there are times when decisions have to be made quickly and if you are not there, then someone else is going to have to make those decisions. There isn't always time to call you. It also generally increases your costs too, because you will need lawyers to assist with the legal filings in two states and there will obviously also be other costs associated with the necessary back and forth flights, although we had no idea the extent to which our costs would increase as a result of what we ultimately ended up experiencing.

There is also another issue though that we did not consider at all and that is the issue of culture, beliefs, and views on surrogacy in the state or country where your surrogacy is located. Because we live in the very liberal state of California, this was again another issue that was not on our radar at all. Surrogacy is not really a thing that anyone bothers about here. It is just viewed as a natural part of the process to become a parent for some people – something that is readily available for those who need it or want to utilize it. Boy, were we in for some shocks though and we learnt this lesson the hard way throughout our journey, but I will tell you more about that soon.

We jumped into the idea of an immediate match with a surrogate because we were so desperate to find a way, any way to start our family and so I don't know if it would have mattered what the agency had said at that time. I think we would have proceeded, nonetheless. The agency told us they had a surrogate who was located in Texas, who had recently completed the screening process and was keen to start the matching process, so they asked if we were interested in meeting her. The surrogate gets the ultimate say in whether or not they would like to meet intended parents.

To determine this, what typically happens is the intended parents are required to create a detailed profile complete with information about your story, your family, your background etc. Pictures are also included so the surrogate and her spouse or partner can get a good sense of who you are and determine whether it might be a good match. This is crucial because it is one of the most important relationships you will ever have in your life – the relationship between the intended parents and the surrogate. For about a year you embark on one of the most intimate relationships of your life. There has to be mutual respect and complete trust in each other and that, as I discovered later, is incredibly difficult to achieve and poses real challenges at times. Dave and I spent a long time developing our intended parents' profile, so that we were best placed to attract a surrogate who would want to work with us. We were thrilled when the agency told us the next day that Monica[11] had confirmed that she

---

11. Name has been changed for privacy/legal reasons

too would like to meet with us. Everything moved quite quickly from that point onwards. A call was scheduled with Monica, her husband, the agency and Dave and I for the following evening. The call went for just over two hours, and we all seemed to get along really well. Generally, after the first meeting call, both the intended parents and the surrogate go away and think about whether they would like to proceed to the next step of an in-person meeting. However, during the call, Monica said that she was happy to meet in person if we would like to do so and we agreed.

The call was on a Wednesday evening, and we arranged to fly to Dallas two days later on the Friday. We decided to make the most of the trip and stay the weekend to sightsee, as Texas had always been a place that we had enjoyed visiting (and eating our way around – great BBQ!). We met with Monica and her husband for lunch on the Friday and while it was clear that we were all very different people, we seemed to get along quite well. I didn't think that Monica and her husband were people that we might otherwise have been friends with, but that didn't matter to me at the time. I wasn't there to make a friend, I was there to find a person who I could work with and trust to carry our child for us, and after both the phone meeting and the in-person meeting, Dave and I felt confident enough that Monica was the right to person to do that for us.

It was also clear that Monica was a 'no-frills' kind of woman. She was clearly hard-working and led a simple life and I respected that. She had also told us she wanted to be a surrogate for two reasons. Firstly, she had watched one of her friends experience fertility issues and she had seen the heartache she had gone through, so she wanted to be able to help another family who was experiencing similar issues as she had not been in the right stage of her life to be able to help her friend at that time. Since then, she had had a daughter of her own and so she was now able to consider doing this for someone else. She also told us that the other reason why she wanted to become a surrogate was so that she could buy a car and take her daughter to Disneyland. I respected and admired her for that.

Monica was part of a low-income family. She lived in a perfectly nice house in Plano, Texas, but there were several members of her husband's extended family living with them and it was clear that they all largely relied on Monica's income to meet the daily financial needs of the household, so there was little room for extras, such as expensive family vacations and trips to theme parks. I respected Monica for being honest with us about her reasons and I thought that was admirable of her to want to provide that kind of wonderful experience for her daughter, so we had no hesitations in proceeding. We flew home from Texas on the Sunday evening feeling happy and full of hope for the first time, in a long time.

The surrogacy agency was notified that we all wanted to proceed and then arrangements were made for Monica to start the process with an IVF doctor in Texas. We also needed to fly to Texas to meet with the doctor who would be assisting us with the embryo transfer there. We had toyed with the idea of flying Monica to L.A. to do the transfer with Dr. Wambach, but we ultimately decided against it. After my experience losing our baby on the flight from Australia, I was nervous about taking that type of risk again with our surrogate. Our little embryos therefore had to be transferred from the lab in L.A. to the doctor in Texas. They are transported in a little freezer and the whole process is not cheap. Another cost that we didn't actually anticipate before deciding to match with a surrogate in another state.

The embryos made it to Texas safely though, and after about two months, Monica was finally ready to do the transfer. There is always some time between the match and the ultimate transfer, because a number of steps need to occur before the transfer can take place. Firstly, there are agreements to be prepared and signed, money to be paid into escrow accounts, documents to be filed in court and various tests to be undertaken on both the intended parents and the surrogate. The surrogate also needs to wait until she is at the right stage of her cycle to be able to undergo the transfer procedure. The doctor will prescribe a contraceptive pill for the month before and a number of pre-natal vitamins so that there are no surprises, and the body is best prepared to accept the embryos.

Unfortunately, neither Dave nor I were able to be in Texas on the day of transfer, something that I will always regret. We both had work commitments that we could not move, and because the timing of the transfer must be so precise, there was no way around it. We were sent lots of pictures though and were so thrilled to see that one of our little embryos was 'hatching' from the zona pellucida (protective shell) on the day of transfer, which was a really good sign!

We only had female embryos left after my unsuccessful transfer, but we decided to implant two embryos, nonetheless. We knew that there would be about a 60 percent chance of at least one baby and about 27 percent chance of twins. Dr. Wambach was quite open-minded when it came to the number of embryos to be transferred at once. The doctor in Texas was less so. It took a lot of convincing before he would agree to transfer two embryos for us. He explained to us that his wife had almost died due to twins and multiple pregnancies carried much higher risk. We really wanted to ensure that we had two chances and we also knew we might not get another chance because of the significant cost associated with surrogacy. In the end, Dr. Wambach managed to convince the doctor in Texas for us and so our two little girls were transferred into Monica's cervix that day.

While Monica was preparing her body for the transfer, I was going through another round of IVF. Because we would only have one embryo left if the transfer with Monica did not work, we wanted to be prepared with more embryos if needed. Therefore, once again I had to put my poor body through the grueling IVF process. We ended up with a large number of eggs again and after the full process through to genetic testing we had five left – all female again.

The next part of the process is excruciating because there is absolutely nothing you can do but wait and hope. You don't want to keep bothering the surrogate because you want her to be calm and relaxed to give your little ones the best possible chance of implanting into their new home. To distract ourselves, we went to the gym a lot and I devoured many, many books on surrogacy and how to create a good relationship with your surrogate. I read lots and lots of amazing stories about surrogates and intended parents from all over the world and we tried to look after Monica well. We would send her little gifts, vitamins, books and many other things to take care of her, and also to let her know how much we appreciated what she was doing for us.

After weeks of waiting and things progressing well, we finally made it to a stage where we could successfully say we were pregnant with not just one, but two of our little babies! I could not wait to tell the world, and on January 4, 2017, we announced it to our friends and family – we had twin baby girls on the way!

After the transfer, things changed. I didn't want to bother Monica all the time for updates, even though the surrogacy agreement clearly says the surrogate is required to provide regular updates, but I found that even checking in once a week would often generate no response from Monica, and we were finding it difficult to get her to communicate about legal documents that had to be signed and other decisions that had to be made. The agency had to step in and intervene a number of times because the communication was so bad. There were two occasions where Monica went to hospital with bleeding and didn't even tell us until days later, in passing comments in text messages. We were so hurt and angry that this was happening. We had believed that Monica was doing this for the right reasons and that she would be everything that we had hoped for in a surrogate, but it became clear that was not the case.

I tried to ask Monica to please just provide me with an update once a week and to let us know immediately if anything like that happened again, but time went on and still the situation did not improve. It was so incredibly hard. I was missing out on the experience of watching the babies grow and develop. I would never feel them move in my stomach or watch their little impressions kick into my belly from within. I was never going to experience any of those things myself, and now Monica was preventing me from experiencing them as our surrogate, even though she was legally supposed to do so. I felt once again cheated and so very sad. Most of the time I had no idea what was going on and at one point Monica made it clear to me (through the agency) that if she felt stressed by the situation, then her doctor was prepared to provide a medical opinion that it was best for her health if we did not communicate. That was crushing. It left us with little choice but to accept the situation and hope and pray for the best. Monica had all of the power and we could do nothing.

The terms of the surrogacy agreement dictate that Monica has the right to select the OBGYN and the hospital, provided that both meet certain requirements. The first one that Monica selected was absolutely awful. I will never forget the day we went for the first appointment and scan. My mother had flown over from Australia, and she was with Dave and I in Texas for that appointment, so there were a lot of people in the room for the scan because Monica, her mother-in-law and her daughter were also there. When the doctor walked into the room he announced, "Why are there so many people in here?" He was clearly annoyed and acted as though he had no idea that it was a surrogacy arrangement. This was not the case, because the agency is heavily involved throughout the entire process and one of the benefits of engaging an agency to assist you is that they always contact the various medical providers and hospitals before a visit, to ensure they are aware of the surrogacy situation, and they have all of the necessary legal documents. This is important because there are privacy laws in play when it comes to the disclosure of medical information, so the doctors and hospitals need to know that they have the legal right to discuss medical information with the intended parents.

In that appointment, the doctor refused to look at Dave, my mother or me. In fact, he refused to address us or acknowledge that we were there at all. At one point when I asked him a question he responded with, "Excuse me, I am talking to the mother" and continued addressing Monica. He then said, "One of the babies is very small. It is unlikely to make it." Just like that! There was no sympathy, no compassion and definitely no care in his delivery at all. I was floored. I started to cry, and he said something along the lines of, "It is what it is. Multiple pregnancies are high risk. There isn't a lot that we can do. Monica, you will need to come back in about a week and we will see if the baby survives."

No way was I going to accept that response. I had been down this road before with my own pregnancy. I immediately walked out and phoned the agency to assist. We wanted another doctor – ASAP! We needed a second opinion and we needed someone who clearly was not opposed to surrogacy and who would be caring and understanding of our situation. Thankfully, the agency agreed, and they told Monica that she had no option. A new doctor was required. So, we all agreed that day to see another doctor the following day for a second opinion.

The second doctor was lovely, and it was a completely different experience. He was much older and wiser and made us feel a lot more at ease. He told us that Baby B was indeed smaller, but that it was common with twins as there is always a dominant one. He told us not to worry just yet, that he would monitor the babies closely. He told Monica she would need to come back for scans regularly for a little while so he could watch the babies' growth. He also told us there were a few things that could be done if it became necessary, but at that stage he just wanted to monitor them. The following day we had no option but to return home to L.A. and this was another example of a situation where I really felt how difficult it was having a surrogate in another state. Because you are not physically carrying a baby yourself, people don't have sympathy in the same way. You are not sick personally, so you don't feel like you can ask for time off work, even though it is needed. I had to return to L.A. and rely on updates from the doctor, because I couldn't rely on Monica to provide them. It was an incredibly stressful situation, which no doubt continued to contribute to my health issues.

Thankfully the babies continued to grow. Baby B ended up getting the nutrients she needed and we were told we were out of the danger zone. I travelled back to Texas a few times over the following weeks for scans and appointments and these were virtually the only updates that we received. I had come to terms with that. It was sad, but there was nothing I could do. It also meant things were awkward between Monica and I when we did see each other at those appointments, and I was starting to feel as though she really disliked me. Dave believes Monica's behavior was driven by jealousy, as Dave and I had a good life. We were happy, we travelled the world for work and had experienced success in our careers, which is everything Monica wanted for her own life. Maybe he is right. I don't know. Whatever it was, it was hurtful, and it was hard, and I found myself longing for it all to be over. All I wanted was to reach the day when we could hold our babies in our arms. Little did we know things were about to get a lot worse.

After two years of treatments, tests, and surgeries I had reached a point where I really wanted to have a hysterectomy. My doctor had told me that while a hysterectomy wasn't a guaranteed cure for endometriosis, in some cases it did help to manage the symptoms. I was so exhausted and sick of being sick, so I decided it was what I wanted. However, Dave really wanted to be able to try for a boy in the future and given that our health insurance plan covered three rounds of IVF, he asked me to undergo one final round. I wasn't keen at all. It had been so hard on my body and had made me so sick and I felt as though we were so lucky to have twin baby girls on the way that I didn't see the need. I didn't want to disappoint Dave though and I knew that he was right. Once I had a hysterectomy, things would change and if I ended up having my ovaries removed, then we would no longer have the option. So I agreed, but only on the basis that this time I would do it as if I didn't care about the outcome.

I was not going to make it a job. I was not going to stop drinking coffee. I was not going to do acupuncture. I was going to live my life as close to normal as I possibly could and see what happened. This third round was therefore not nearly as difficult for me, and I found I wasn't as unwell as I had been the first two times. I realized one of the reasons why I had been so sick was because I had cut out all caffeine and this had contributed to my awful migraines. This time, I did not stop drinking coffee and the migraines were not nearly as bad. I got through it and by the end we had another three female embryos and one male. Clearly Dave's male sperm cannot swim!

A week later I was back in hospital, but this time it was to have a hysterectomy and I can honestly tell you it was the best decision I have ever made in my life. Did it cure my endometriosis? No. But it did change my life. I had lived for almost twenty years with such heavy bleeding, discomfort, and pain, that I would have to change my clothes multiple times a day. I cannot tell you how many times I would wake up in the night with blood soaked through my mattress or how many days I would leak through my clothes when out in public, but for me, even worse were the migraines. Since I was a little girl, I have had debilitating migraines at least four or five times a week. Honestly, they were so bad that it really was a disability in and of itself.

My grandmother and my mother have lived their lives just the same, as they too have suffered from awful migraines. I also know my grandmother had menstrual issues and pregnancy losses and I wonder whether she too may have had endometriosis as well. It wasn't something that was known at all back then, but she did have a hysterectomy in her early fifties and her migraines stopped, so it would not surprise me at all if she suffered from it as well.

Hysterectomies aren't miracles for everyone and sometimes they end up causing people more problems than they had before the procedure, so I am definitely not here to advocate that it is something that everyone should do. However, for me it changed my life in a really positive way. I was never able to really enjoy exercise because I was constantly suffering from migraines. Every three weeks I would bleed so much that even leaving the house was difficult at times, let alone attempting something like exercise! I am not saying I never get migraines now, because I do, but they are significantly less than before. Whereas I previously suffered from migraines at least four or five times a week, I now only get them two or three times a month if that. For me, that is a significant improvement. I also never again have to worry about wearing white clothes, wearing a maternity pad, two pairs of underwear and shorts under pants or a dress. I no longer have to worry about making sure I never leave the house without a bag packed full of spare underwear, pants and pads. I feel free for the first time since I was twelve.

There are certain things that happen when you have a hysterectomy. Firstly, it is a major surgery because you are having organs removed, so there is going to be some recovery time. There are emotional side effects as well that I didn't quite expect, given that I was all for the procedure. You also do feel a bit different down there because your uterus, cervix, fallopian tubes and possibly one or both of your ovaries are now missing. I did feel a little hollow and I am not ashamed to say that I can no longer sneeze or jump on the trampoline without wetting myself just a little, but for me that is all fine, albeit slightly annoying. I wouldn't hesitate to do it again. It's one of the best decisions that I have ever made for myself.

The day after my hysterectomy I was in the hospital recovering. Dave was there with me visiting when his phone rang. It was a doctor at a hospital in Texas. Monica had selected the hospital where she wanted to deliver the babies. It wasn't the one we would have selected, but I was not going to object, because at least they seemed pleasant enough when we had visited to complete all of the necessary paperwork. It had been an interesting visit though, as they had tried to convince us to let Monica breastfeed the babies after birth and also suggested that we might like to be in the water with Monica as she gave birth to the babies[12] – a suggestion that we both quickly, but politely declined! This call was from a different hospital though and not one that we recognized. It turned out that the hospital that Monica had selected for the delivery did not have an emergency department, so they were only set up to cater for straightforward births without complications.

The doctor on the other end of the call told Dave and I that Monica was in the hospital. She had arrived with bleeding and there were complications, as her cervix was dilated seven centimeters, which meant the babies were at real risk of being born. Monica was only twenty-three weeks' pregnant at this stage, so it was crucial that didn't happen. We were worried sick. The doctor told us the babies would have a five percent chance of survival and asked if we wanted the hospital to attempt resuscitation. When we said yes, she responded rudely: "Do you know what quality of life they would have?", as if we were making the wrong choice. Her manner was completely cold and abrupt, and I will never forget that call for the rest of my life and how cruel the doctor was in her communication with us that day.

I was in no state to be able to travel. Dave didn't want to leave me, and he knew I would need help after I was released from hospital. Through tears I told him that if our babies were going to be born and then pass, I didn't want them to be alone. I wanted to know they would be able to pass away in his arms being wrapped in our love. We had no other option – my mother had to come. Within a few hours, Dave was on a plane to Texas and my mother was on a plane on her way

---

12. Monica had selected a water birth in the hospital. They had large birthing tubs in all of the rooms at this particular hospital.

from Australia to me in L.A. My mother ended up staying in the U.S. for five weeks to help us. She was a saint during that time. We could not have done it without her because those days were really, really tough. They were the hardest days I have ever experienced in my life and every single hour is precious during a high-risk pregnancy when there is a high chance of premature birth. You find yourself hoping and praying every minute that passes that the babies will stay where they are just a little bit longer.

We were told sometime later that our surrogate's cervix had closed, and the contractions had stopped, but that Monica was to be placed on strict bed rest in the hospital where she would be monitored by a team of doctors, including a perinatologist, due to the high-risk nature of the pregnancy. The perinatologist later told us she did not believe that the cervix actually was dilated seven centimeters at all, but that we had been told this in error.

We didn't want to miss any call or update, so we decided Dave would need to remain in Texas until I could travel. So, while Dave was in Texas with Monica, I was in L.A with my mother until about ten days later when I was well enough to travel. I was swollen and sore, so we didn't want to risk plane travel. My poor mother therefore had to drive the two of us all the way from L.A. to Dallas. We did it with just one overnight stop on the way, and not without some drama to boot. In the stress of the situation, and given that we were not travelling by air, I had accidentally forgotten my passport. Going through Texas near the border of Mexico means that you encounter a border control checkpoint. When we were stopped and I was unable to produce my passport, I ended up in trouble.

The border control officer said I would have to go to the camp for further processing until the matter could be resolved. I was terrified. I needed to get to Texas in case my babies were born, which could be at any minute. I couldn't afford this delay and I was also still very unwell. I had only just had major surgery about ten days prior, so I certainly didn't want to end up locked up in a camp where I wouldn't be able to rest or have access to the medications I needed. Not to mention I was still working solidly throughout, and I wasn't sure what on earth would happen to my workload if I was locked up and unable to access my laptop or emails.

Just as I was about to be carted away, while my mother was screaming at me from the car to hand over my jewelry so that I didn't get robbed, I suddenly remembered I might have a picture of my work visa on my phone, as I recalled taking a picture of it to send a copy to our firm's immigration team. I asked the border control officers if they would permit me to look in my phone to see if I had a copy and they agreed. Thankfully I found it and they agreed to issue me with a written warning this time, but ultimately did let me go. I learnt a very good lesson that day. There is no leniency. If you're travelling in the U.S. as a non-citizen, you must have your passport with you.

We continued on our journey and reached Texas two days later, both exhausted from the journey, but anxious to see our babies on the scan. I was relieved when the doctors told us things were looking much better and they hoped that Monica would be able to hold on for quite a few more weeks yet. We finally had some comfort and relief, so Dave headed back to L.A. for work while my mother and I remained in Texas. We ended up having to rent an apartment in Texas because it had become clear that our great plan to fly in and out and then collect the babies after birth and return home within a few days was not going to happen. Whether we liked it or not, Texas was to be our home away from home for the foreseeable future. It also meant Dave and I would be forced to spend many weeks apart, because while I had complete flexibility to work remotely, Dave was not so fortunate, and his boss was not very understanding of our situation. On numerous occasions in those early weeks, he told Dave he would have to get back to L.A. or he would no longer have a job. Needless to say, as soon as Dave was able to do so, he moved on to a better company.

My mother stayed with me in Texas for a further four weeks before we unfortunately had to say goodbye to her. It was such a sad day. I desperately wanted her to stay. Monica was continuing to be difficult and argumentative with me every day. When Dave was there, she was fine, but when it was her and I on our own it was a real struggle. I have no doubt that those weeks in the hospital were difficult for her, but the whole experience was made worse because of her attitude towards me. I couldn't understand it, and neither could the agency. We did everything we possibly could to try to keep her happy. We arranged for a streaming device in her room, bought her crafts that she requested, arranged for a laptop for her to do a course, had the hospital bring in a fridge, which we kept stocked with her favorite foods and I continued to bring her gifts and flowers to brighten her day. The agency and I also arranged for a hairdresser to come in and do her hair, as she had not been able to get up to shower or wash it. It didn't matter what I did though, Monica continued to be hostile and mean and there was nothing that I could do. I just had to keep going, say nothing and be the better person.

After a few weeks in the hospital, as things had started to become less of a crisis, Monica had made it clear she did not want to be in the hospital on bed rest until she reached term. I don't blame her. It was an awful situation, but the fact is that when you decide to become a surrogate, you know the risks. You are made well aware of your obligations, and you have human life, or in our case, lives in your hands, so regardless of how uncomfortable or awful the situation is, the needs of the babies must come first, unless it poses a risk to the life of the surrogate. There are certainly cases where surrogates have had to abort or deliver early where the pregnancy has posed a risk to their own life, and I am certainly not suggesting in those cases that the life of the surrogate should be secondary to the needs of the child. In those types of situations there is absolutely a justification for putting the needs of the babies second. However, that was not our situation.

Yes, it was awful that Monica had to be in hospital on bed rest for so many weeks. No, it is certainly not the experience I would have wanted for her or for us, but it was unfortunately how it all played out. We did our very best to make sure Monica was as comfortable as possible and had everything she needed and wanted during that time, so that the experience was bearable for her. One of the conditions under the surrogacy agreement is that if your surrogate cannot work at any point during the pregnancy you have to pay for her salary, so Monica was certainly not financially disadvantaged in any way as a result of the extended hospital stay. We would have made sure of that anyway, even if it had not been part of the agreement.

The perinatologist[13] was primarily responsible for making the decisions regarding our surrogate and our twins and this was evidenced by the fact that I would often ask the doctor if Monica was able to get up to take a shower or use the toilet, as we knew that this was something that she really wanted to be able to do. On each occasion the doctor would comment, "Not until we check with the perinatologist". The head doctor of the ward repeated the message from the perinatologist, that under no circumstances should our surrogate get up.

Although we had rented an apartment and committed to staying in Texas until the birth of our children, on April 30, 2017, I unfortunately had to fly back to Los Angeles as I had a work commitment that I could not miss. I had planned to only be gone two days. Dave was also back in Los Angeles for work at that time and had been flying back in on weekends. On the morning of April 30, before I left Texas, I went into the hospital to see Monica. I had been told the day before that the perinatologist would be attending that morning to do a scan, so I also wanted to be there for that before I flew out.

During that session with the perinatologist, I became so distressed as a result of being ignored by the doctor that I yelled: "They are my babies! Can you please speak to me?" The doctor made me feel as though I had no business being in the room that day, as she had placed the monitor directly in my line of view with her back to me. She was speaking softly to Monica about "her babies", refusing to acknowledge that I was actually their mother. Unfortunately, this was not an isolated incident and was typical of the type of behavior that Dave and I were subjected to by numerous staff at the hospital.

During that visit, our surrogate once again asked the perinatologist if she was now able to get up out of bed to use the toilet and shower, given that she was now twenty-eight weeks into the pregnancy. The perinatologist responded in a firm manner.

---

13. Maternal–fetal medicine, also known as perinatology, is a branch of medicine that focuses on managing health concerns of the mother and fetus prior to, during, and shortly after pregnancy. Maternal–fetal medicine specialists are physicians who subspecialize within the field of obstetrics.

"Absolutely not! If you get up those babies will come immediately."

There was another thing about that visit with Monica on April 30 that would end up haunting me. It was the last time I ever saw Monica, and my last memory of her before I left the hospital room was of her saying to me, "I have Googled it and the babies are now twenty-eight weeks, so they can survive on their own". Those words traumatized me in the days and weeks that followed. Maybe I could have changed things if I hadn't flown back to LA. I will never know.

After the perinatologist had concluded her examination, I left the hospital feeling terribly upset. I cried all the way to the airport and called Dave on the way to tell him that I did not know how much more I could take of being treated like this.

Later that evening when I was back at home in Los Angeles, I was looking at Facebook and noticed that our surrogate had posted a message saying: "Yay! Just got up to have my first shower in five weeks. Feels amazing!" Dave and I immediately called the hospital in distress to find out why our surrogate had been permitted to get up and have a shower when the perinatologist's instructions just that morning had been so clear. The hospital advised us that there had been a junior doctor on staff that evening who clearly had not known about the previous instructions. We were told that our surrogate asked her if she could get up, and the doctor agreed.

We asked whether she had read the file notes or consulted with the perinatologist and were told that she had not done so. Sometime later that evening, Dave received a call directly from the doctor in question who told him that she didn't even know we were the parents, and that Monica was a surrogate. The hospital was well aware of the surrogacy arrangement. All of the required legal documents had been sent to the hospital administration the day that our surrogate was admitted into hospital. It is something that the agency takes care of, and they had assured us that it had been done. There was no excuse for this. It was pure negligence, and it was completely unacceptable.

We don't know how long our surrogate would have remained with our twins in utero, but what we do know for a fact is that when we were at the hospital, there were absolutely no signs the babies were coming on that day. There were no signs of distress and no signs that labor was imminent. We also know that the perinatologist had unequivocally stated that if our surrogate got up, the babies would come. Additionally, the junior doctor on that night shift did not seek the opinion of the treating perinatologist before she made a terribly negligent decision. It is also undisputed that every single day in utero counts when babies are this young gestationally and that even another few days or a week or a few weeks could have made a world of difference for our children.

Despite many attempts, we have never been given any satisfactory response as to how or why this negligence occurred, but ultimately it resulted in our surrogate commencing labor within minutes after the shower occurred and the birth of our twins the next day. Even worse though, is that this is something we were not even advised of until many hours after the twins had been born (we received a call at 3.43pm on May 1) and we later discovered our surrogate was actually in labor when we were on the phone to the hospital about the shower incident the previous evening. But no one bothered to tell us and therefore we were denied the opportunity to try to get to Dallas for their birth.

The whole situation caused Dave and I both a considerable amount of distress. We had waited so long for this and we could very well have been there, had the hospital done the right thing and told us the evening before that Monica was in labor. Even worse though for me was the fact that our babies were lying on their own in the NICU for so many hours before we were notified and given the opportunity to get there. There were multiple opportunities for the hospital to let us know about the labor and they did not do so. We had two phone calls with hospital staff and doctors on the evening of April 30 whilst our surrogate was in labor and not one person ever mentioned it. We also had another phone call with the head doctor on the morning of May 1 and he did not say a word about our surrogate being in labor either. Had we been told when she entered labor, we would not have missed the birth of our children. Instead, we received a call from the hospital over two hours after the twins' birth to tell us that they had been born and were fighting for their lives in the NICU.

During those five weeks leading up to the twins' birth, the treatment that both Dave and I were subjected to by hospital staff was absolutely appalling. We were never consulted about the status of our twins and decisions that were made for them without our knowledge or consent. Frequently, doctors would come to review our surrogate and take scans of our babies and we were treated as if we were not even in the room.

As people who had lost four babies and had gone through an extremely complex, painful, and lengthy process to be able to have our twins, to have been subjected to this kind of treatment from the hospital staff was absolutely heartbreaking. We had every right to be consulted, given up-to-date information and to be treated with dignity and respect, and not once did I personally feel I was given that courtesy. We were undergoing what was an incredibly stressful time, as we did not know from one day to the next whether our little girls were going to survive and if they did, what quality of life they would ultimately have.

We arrived at the hospital at 2 a.m. on the second of May, 2017. We saw our babies for the first time, and we wept. We were not allowed to hold them. Being that little, they were in a temperature regulated incubator in the NICU. We were able to put our hands in through two holes though to touch them and I was able to hold their little hands – so, so tiny. Babies born that prematurely are stressed anyway, so we were told we would have to be very careful. The nurses told us not to stroke them or do anything other than a light, solid touch. I couldn't believe I was actually a mother. After all of the years of heartache, I had two tiny, little babies. They were so very small, but so very precious. I loved them instantly. It was like I'd been struck by lightning.

We stayed in the hospital with them, learning from the nurses everything we could about them, what their issues were and what they needed. We were told that Twin A (Savannah) was strong. She was just tiny and needed time to grow, but otherwise they did not have any concerns about her. Twin B (Adaline) was a different story. She was tiny and feisty. This posed a problem because she moved around and cried so much that she was losing too much weight, but there were other issues for poor little Adi too. She had two holes in her heart and a bleed on her brain. She also had difficulties breathing, which required oxygen. Adi was going to need a lot of care and prayer to make it and while Dave and I continually swapped positions in the NICU so that we both had time with each baby, I did focus more of my time on little Adi in those days. I was so desperate for her to hold on and I know that she needed me more.

About ten days later, we were finally able to hold our babies for the first time and it is still the most special memory I hold in my heart to this day. There is no better feeling in life than the moment when you get to hold your child in your arms for the first time, and words will never really do justice to how special a moment that really is. It is something that I will close my eyes and be able to remember for the rest of my life. When I look at our little girls now, as they are about to turn four, I can still remember that feeling and I cannot believe how far they have come from those tiny little babies that lay on our bare chests that day. Adi was especially so very, very tiny. She has always been tiny and is still. I call her my little poppet. Our main focus was the babies' survival, but I was also full of rage and there is no telling what I would have done to Monica had I ever seen her in those days following the girls' birth. They were so very tiny and frail, and they had many incredibly difficult days ahead of them between birth and when they were finally released from the hospital three-and-a-half months' later. I know we were incredibly lucky. I can sit here now writing this in the knowledge that our children are okay, and we are truly blessed, because not everyone is nearly that fortunate. People lose babies every day and premature babies pass away in the NICU every day too.

At the time, we had no idea whether our little ones were going to survive and all I knew was that this woman had failed us, and more importantly, she had failed our children. I was so full of sadness and rage in those early days after the babies were born and I knew that if I saw her, I couldn't trust myself not to do something that I would end up regretting. We told the hospital that Monica wasn't allowed to come near us or the babies ever again. It was so unfortunate that our journey had to end like this, but honestly given the way Monica had acted throughout the pregnancy anyway and her animosity towards me, I wasn't sure we would have ended up with a relationship after the birth anyway. Maybe Monica thought it would be easier for her that way as well. I guess we will never know what her motivations really were. I will never understand what went wrong in our surrogacy journey and I am saddened by the experience that we ultimately had. Monica's attitude had been terrible right throughout the pregnancy. The agency did try to assist us throughout the process, but they too had challenges dealing with Monica. They told us later that they had never had such a difficult surrogate. It had caused so much stress for us and my own health suffered as a result. It was an emotional and difficult time and not at all what I had imagined it would be like. At the end of the day, we have two beautiful children and with time you learn to forget, and focus on just the good that came out of the experience – the fact that we have two amazing little humans because they are all that matters! Unfortunately, the girls' condition wasn't the only stress we had to deal with during the days and weeks after they were born. There was issue after issue with the hospital. They had complied with our wishes and ensured that Monica was not granted access to the babies though, which is one of the only things that I cannot fault them on.

As Monica was recovering from a cesarean she remained in the hospital for a few days after the birth, but they had moved her to a completely separate area of the hospital so that there would be little chance of us running into any of her family members, or Monica herself, upon her departure. I was grateful for that at least, but unfortunately it was not characteristic of the rest of the treatment that we would be subjected to by the hospital in the weeks that followed. During that time, we suffered from hostility, incompetence and dishonesty. Texas is unlike California in that there is a very large degree of cultural conservatism, in some cases based on religion.

We were amazed and perplexed at how openly hostile so many of the medical providers were to us in Texas because our children had been born via surrogate. It may have been counter to the published policies of the hospital, but as the American saying goes, culture eats policy for lunch every time. But the worst things we were confronted with were the incompetence and the dishonesty.

Getting Home

As the twins grew stronger, we started to enquire about the possibility of having them transferred to a hospital closer to our home in Los Angeles. We spoke to one of the doctors about it as well, as the twins' pediatrician back in L.A. and the hospital that we wanted to transfer them to, and they were all of the view that the twins had reached a point where transportation would be safe provided it was done via air ambulance.

By late May 2017, the treating doctor at the hospital had given authorization for the twins to be transported by air ambulance to a Los Angeles hospital. However, what transpired over the next few weeks was nothing short of unbelievable.

We were fully aware that the only way to have any hope of getting the twins out of the hospital would be if we paid for the cost of transportation, something that we were absolutely prepared to do. We were desperate to get the twins out of the hospital because after what had happened surrounding their birth, we had absolutely no faith in the care that they were being provided. In addition, we had real concerns about some of the treatments that our twins were being subjected to (more on that later).

Despite the doctor's medical clearance, we received pushbacks and rejections from the hospital. We were constantly lied to and obstacle after obstacle was placed in our way in an attempt to block us from having the twins' transported. On at least three occasions we were told by the hospital in Los Angeles that they were ready and willing to accept the twins and that they had sent the authorization to accept them, and on each occasion, we were lied to by the hospital staff and told they had not received the authorization. Even our health insurance company told us they had sent through the authorizations. They also told us it is illegal to withhold the release of babies, pending receipt of authorizations from a health insurance company. Things got so bad that the insurance company ended up advising us to call the police and report the hospital for kidnapping.

We were also forced to use First Flight, an air ambulance transportation company we were told was the only company that the hospital would approve for the transfer of the girls, despite the fact that it was the most expensive transportation option. Both St. John's and UCLA hospitals in Santa Monica had their own transportation services which were cheaper, and representatives from both hospitals advised us that they could highly recommend the services, as they frequently used them to transfer patients, including NICU babies. Both of their services would have also used NICU trained nurses for the transport of the babies via air ambulance. Nonetheless, the hospital would not accept this and forced us to use First Flight. We were told that unless we used this service then they would not allow the girls to leave the hospital.

As such, we paid $27,750 to First Flight on May 31, 2017. First Flight notified us they were ready and able to transport the twins the next day. On at least five occasions over the next two weeks, we were told by First Flight they were ready and able to transport the twins the next day and on every single occasion the hospital blocked the transfer, telling us that First Flight was not able to do the transfer. Each time we would again go back to First Flight to confirm this, and they would repeat the same message to us, that the hospital staff had specifically told them to stall us. Time and time again we were continually lied to. Months later, First Flight actually contacted us to ask us if we intended to take legal action against the hospital as they had just assumed that we would in light of the treatment that we were subjected to.

After weeks of stress and anxiety trying desperately to get our children home, so that we could finally be surrounded by friends and our support network, we had reached a point where we were desperate. On June 1, 2017, we had a meeting with the hospital's legal team and unbelievably, during that meeting not only did the hospital representatives continue to deny that they were deliberately blocking the transfer, even though the emails from First Flight clearly proved this, but they also threatened to call Child Services to report us if we attempted to transfer our children to UCLA.

There was absolutely no basis whatsoever for the hospital to make such a threat to two loving parents. We had done everything the hospital had asked of us and more, and at no time were we ever putting the lives of our children at risk. The hospital doctors had agreed the twins were safe to travel, we had a world-class hospital lined up to take the girls, the doctors at UCLA had reviewed the twins' medical records, had beds set up and had told us they had increased nursing staff numbers to accommodate the transfer. We had also agreed and paid for the transportation company that the hospital had demanded we use, and yet after all of this our attempts were met with a threat to report us for absolutely no reason. The hospital's actions were absolutely disgusting and shameful.

It was only after we threatened legal action, and that we had been told by our insurance company to call the police, that we were finally able to have the twins transferred to UCLA hospital in Santa Monica, California. To say that our experience at UCLA was different is an understatement. The treatment and care that Savannah and Adaline, Dave and I received was like night and day compared to what we had experienced at the hospital in Texas.

From the minute that we arrived at UCLA, there was never any question around our parentage of the twins. The twins received excellent care at UCLA, and they made it very clear from day one that it was their aim to release the twins as soon as possible. In fact, they surprised even us as Savannah only ended up having to be at UCLA for an additional two and a half weeks and Adaline four and a half weeks. We have no doubt at all that had our girls been forced to remain at the hospital in Texas they would have stayed in the NICU for a much longer period.

When the doctors and nurses at UCLA reviewed the twins' medical records and we told them further information about the treatments that had been provided to the twins at the hospital in Texas, they were shocked. The twins had been forced to wear a C-Pap[14] until they reached 32 weeks. UCLA told us that the C-Pap is such outdated technology that they have not used it in the NICU there for about ten years. They said it causes such stress to the premature infants that

---

14. Continuous positive airway pressure is a form of positive airway pressure ventilation in which a constant level of pressure greater than atmospheric pressure is continuously applied to the upper respiratory tract of a person

it delays their development and can cause health issues. Whilst I was not aware of this when the twins were at the hospital in Texas, I did feel very unhappy with the C-Pap, especially because Savannah had virtually no breathing issues after the first couple of days post-birth. I constantly fought with doctors and nursing staff at the hospital about the need for Savannah, in particular, to have to wear the C-Pap and was repeatedly told that it was absolutely needed and that if I took it off the children, I would be reported to the hospital's security.

The reason why we were so concerned about the C-Pap ourselves is that the girls were clearly in distress almost the entire time they were forced to wear it. They both cried constantly when forced to wear nasal prongs, it caused damage to their face and nose, and they were clearly incredibly uncomfortable. We have no doubt that this impacted their development and growth because the agitation caused weight loss for many weeks post-birth.

During our time at both the hospital in Texas and at UCLA we were told that their policies were that a child had to have five days clear of any recorded incidents before they were eligible for release from the NICU. An incident is a recordable 'brady' or d-saturation. For an incident to be recordable, the heart rate or oxygen level has to fall below a certain number. During our time in the NICU at the hospital in Texas loud, obnoxious alarms were constantly going off to alert the nursing staff and doctors to a 'recordable incident'. The longer a baby continues to have recordable incidents, the longer the baby must remain in the NICU and therefore the better it is for the hospital financially.

We are well aware of the payment that the hospital would receive for each day that a child remains in the NICU, and we believe that this was also the reason why we experienced such horrific measures to prevent us from transferring the children to UCLA. We had no reason to believe that the alarms were anything but normal practice until we reached UCLA. At UCLA the alarms were a lot quieter. Again, they told us that this was to avoid startling the babies and causing them unnecessary stress, which is critical to their growth and development. Not only did the high alarming thresholds and high volumes distress the babies, but it completely distressed us as parents witnessing it.

Additionally, once we got to UCLA, we noted something much more serious that had clearly been happening at the hospital in Texas. It became clear to us very quickly that what the hospital does is set the levels to such a high state, whereby a baby's heart rate or oxygen level only needs to drop by a very small amount to trigger the loud alarms and generate a recordable incident. By doing this it justifies the hospital keeping the babies in the NICU for much longer periods. In fact, when we inquired of many of the nurses at the hospital in Texas as to what the average gestational age is when babies are released from the NICU there, they informed us that babies rarely leave before full-term and some even stay post-term. They told us not to expect to be able to leave for quite some time.

In contrast, as soon as we arrived at UCLA and they had an opportunity to observe the twins, they told us they didn't anticipate they would need very much longer in the NICU, which turned out to be correct. UCLA told us their objective is to get babies home as quickly as reasonably possible and that babies rarely stay in the NICU to term unless they were born micro-preemies (a baby born before twenty-six weeks gestation, or who weigh less than one pound, twelve ounces).

It was also clear to both Dave and me when our children were in the NICU at the hospital in Texas, that the hospital staff were displeased with how much time we spent there each day. We were in the hospital between ten and sixteen hours a day every single day and were frequently told, "You spend too much time here. Why don't you go home?" There was nowhere else that we would have even considered being, but with our children. We did not trust the medical advice or care that was being given to our children and frankly we had nowhere else to go. Texas was not our home. However, if you're not there in the hospital as much as we were, then the things that we observed are practices that a parent would probably never pick up. Even before being transferred to UCLA, Dave and I could just sense that things were not right, and we were constantly caused to question the advice we were being given and the treatment methods that were being used on our twins.

The experience we had at the hospital in Texas was nothing short of a nightmare. In addition to all of the problems we had managing our daughters' treatment and trying to get them safely home to California, something else happened to me while we were there. On numerous occasions whilst the twins were in the hospital, when I was doing kangaroo care (skin-to-skin contact with the babies, which is good for their development) with one or both of my daughters, one of the respiratory team members Toby would wait until I was naked from the waist up and even though I would have the hospital curtains drawn around me, he would enter the enclosed area under the premise that he needed to adjust the babies' C-Pap masks at just that time.

He would stand over me leering down my naked chest making me feel terribly uncomfortable. He only ever did it to me, and only ever when Dave was not present, but it happened enough times when I was on my own that I understood exactly what he was doing. I felt completely helpless and violated. I told Dave many times that I wasn't sure what to do about it, but ultimately, we decided we would not make a complaint at that time, as we certainly did not want any negative repercussions for the twins, and they were the priority. Dave and I also witnessed Toby frequently make inappropriate comments of a sexual nature towards the nursing staff and he was often referred to by them as "dirty Toby". Toby made me feel so uncomfortable that I would physically shudder every time I would see him enter the NICU and even writing this after years have passed, I still feel sick thinking back to those times. Needless to say, when our babies were finally wheeled out of that hospital and onto the plane, I burst into tears. We were finally free, and I never had to look back at that place again.

I've never been able to bring myself to go back to Texas since leaving that day with the twins. In the future, I would like to take them back and show them where they were born and tell them the story of their beginning, minus all of the horrible bits of course. I am really thankful that I had written a formal complaint to the Texas Medical Board after we returned to California detailing everything that had happened to us, because I was able to access that document to recall exactly everything that we went through. As I read back through the complaints though, I realized just how much of our story I had blocked out of my mind.

The human body is an amazing organ, and it always fascinates me that our minds have the ability to close off certain painful memories like that for self-preservation. Honestly, going back through it all now though and laying it out in this book, I don't know how we ever got through it all, but I am thankful that I don't feel the same aversion to surrogacy as I do to Texas, as a result of our experience. Rather, I have tried to use our experience in a positive way by assisting to influence much needed change to the law and by providing information and support to other families who are undertaking similar journeys, often following their own heartbreak.

The Fight for Parental Rights

I can honestly tell you that before having our children I knew basically nothing about surrogacy laws in any country. A number of our friends had children born via surrogate, but it wasn't something I never asked them about. I had no reason to pay much attention to any discussion about surrogacy, let alone the legal aspects, until it became a huge and vitally important part of my world. Because we were under so much stress at the time, we decided to enter into a surrogacy arrangement, then after our surrogate was pregnant and of course when they were born premature and had to remain in the hospital, it didn't actually cross our minds to consider the laws in Australia. I think that because surrogacy is so widely accepted in the U.S where we were living and as we had already engaged a lawyer in Texas to handle the legal aspects of the arrangement, we just didn't even consider that we might encounter some challenges if we ever wanted to live in Australia again with our children.

As a lawyer, I read legal updates every single day and in January 2017, I happened to see an article that a lawyer in Brisbane had published, which the Law Institute in Victoria had included in their weekly newsletter. My best friend Sharon, who is a lawyer herself, had also seen it and she sent it to me. It was a particularly troublesome report, and it really was my first insight into the problems that Dave and I were about to experience in our legal battle in Australia.

In the article, the lawyer had outlined the significant issues that exist in Australia regarding surrogacy laws, the challenges that parents of children born via surrogacy were facing to be recognized as the legal parents under Australian law, and the implications of these types of arrangements. These could include issues regarding a parent's right to make medical or schooling decisions, or ensure that their children would hold the legal right to inherit superannuation and other assets upon death. In the article, the lawyer also provided an overview of the law, and outlined the fact that commercial surrogacy arrangements are not legal in Australia and are an offence in three states. I remember reading this article and feeling immediately sick. I honestly had no idea about any of these issues until reading that article and I did what most people would do in those circumstances; I immediately emailed the lawyer to ask if he could assist us. As it happened, I was due to be in Australia for work the following week and so the lawyer agreed to meet with me.

I immediately liked this lawyer as soon as I met with him, and I knew almost instantly he was the right person to assist us. He was clearly extremely knowledgeable about international surrogacy and the legal landscape in Australia, but more importantly, he also had his own experiences to draw from as well. In my view the very best service providers in any field are the ones that can not only speak from an expert point of view, but who can also relate and empathize with the issue on the basis of their lived experiences as well. When you are advising clients on issues that you have personally experienced, you are able to empathize and better understand and anticipate the needs of the client because you know exactly the type of information, advice, and support you also needed at that time. There are thousands of great lawyers, accountants and financial planners on offer, but I really recommend seeking out those with shared experiences, as it is often the difference between a great service provider and an exceptional one.

The lawyer explained to Dave and me that while we would likely be able to obtain Australian citizenship for our children eventually, it was a complex process because of the surrogacy laws in Australia. He also told us we would not hold legal parental rights under Australian law because of the overseas surrogacy arrangement and that our only option was to seek a parental order from the Family Court, which of course was going to end up being costly. At that time, we had planned to move back to Australia in December after the girls were born, so we could be closer to our families. I was incredibly angry and completely worn down, as we were faced with one challenge after the next.

I just wanted us to be able to get on with our lives, but at every turn it seemed like there was another hurdle, another person waiting with a roadblock and a sign that said, "You just wait a minute now. You're still not cleared to pass go!". I felt enraged through both frustration and exhaustion, and I couldn't believe that after all that we had been through, anyone was going to dare try to tell us our children were not our own. Even trying to think objectively, it just didn't make any sense to me. We had strictly followed the law of the country where we were residing, we had followed the required process, they were genetically ours (although in my opinion that should not matter at all) and we had a court order confirming they were legally ours in the United States. I was completely incredulous about these further roadblocks. After everything that we had been through though, I was not about to take any chances. I didn't want this to be an issue in the future for any of us, most importantly the girls, so we immediately hired the lawyer and he set to work on our case.

At the same time as we were engaging in our legal battle in Australia, I was inadvertently becoming an advocate for surrogacy rights in Australia. Our personal situation was certainly distressing but honestly, for me, I was more concerned about the much broader implications of what we had discovered. It felt so unbelievably unjust to me, and it was such a complicated issue that required considerable time and resources to navigate, and I couldn't stop thinking about how these two factors would prohibit most people in Australia who were suffering from fertility issues from utilizing this option. That made me more upset than anything else.

Here I was, an educated lawyer myself and not only a lawyer, but one practicing on a global scale. A large part of my practice involves helping clients to navigate the laws in new markets and cross-border legal issues, so you might say I have some expertise when it comes to complex legal issues involving multiple countries. I was also fortunate enough to be in a situation where I have a lot of legal contacts and I had the resources to be able to access the help we needed. I realized very quickly just how daunting and difficult the whole process would seem without all of these things.

I could picture myself in our old apartment on the day when I found out that our embryo transfer had not worked, hearing my doctor's voice telling me that she didn't think we should try again, and I thought back to how utterly devastated and heartbroken I had felt in that moment. I remembered the tears I had shed that day and how my doctor's suggestion of surrogacy had given me the hope I needed to keep going and to push through to another day. I then imagined what would have happened to me had that not been an option. What if I had never ended up in the U.S. and I had been living in Australia? There is a good chance I would never have even considered surrogacy had I remained there, because it just isn't something that is generally presented as a viable option to consider.

I have now learnt that the legal landscape makes it virtually impossible, unless you have a generous family member or friend that is willing to help you out ex gratia, but those situations are few and far between. What makes the situation even more dire in Australia for those suffering fertility issues is that for most people, adoption is also out of reach. In 2019–2020, there were only three hundred and thirty-four adoptions in Australia and figures have been around this number for many years. Because of the limited availability of children to adopt, couples who would like to adopt can end up waiting years, with many never succeeding.

There are also a number of requirements to qualify for adoption, so it is also not something that is possible for every couple either. Adoption is therefore not the simple solution to fertility struggles that many people believe. Yet comments such as, "Why don't you just adopt?" are frequently heard by people experiencing fertility issues. It is also not something that is right for every couple, it can be a long, difficult and complex process and a big decision for everyone involved.

It is also important to remember there is a child involved who may have experienced trauma, abandonment, neglect and/or abuse. The child is the most important person in the relationship and so a person should only ever consider adoption if they are truly committed to all that it involves, because it could be detrimental to a child to go through an adoption and have it not work out. In our case, Dave was not open to the idea, and I would never force him into something that he was not one hundred percent committed to for that reason. It would not be fair to any party.

Honestly, I am not sure I could have survived the kind of heartbreak that I experienced, were it not for the fact that we had another very real, viable option in surrogacy. The day after Dr. Wambach called me with the news, we had literally started the process by investigating the option and setting up a meeting with the agency. It gave me hope, but it also provided me with the perfect distraction. I was able to get up and keep going. I had a purpose again and I had a newfound determination and will to keep moving forward, but none of that would have happened were it not for the fact that I was living in a country and state where it was possible. And now, after all of that, we found ourselves back in an extremely complex web of legal challenges.

The issue of surrogacy rights and the impact that the harsh Australian laws were having on a lot of families in our situation made me so angry that I felt I had no option but to start speaking up on the issue, which was far bigger than our own situation. I found that the more that I spoke out about the issue, the more I came to realize just how little was known about surrogacy in the community. While some people had heard of it, most people I spoke to didn't really know what it was or what it entailed. Hardly anyone was aware of the legal restrictions that are in place and the fact that engaging in commercial surrogacy is a crime in three Australian states.

Once you put a face and a story to an issue, it generally creates a far different perception for people. If I ever talk about an issue such as surrogacy and just stick to facts, people who have heard of it, but know little about it, tend to relate the issue back to the baby Gammy case[15], or other similar tragic stories of surrogacy gone wrong. And why?

Well for many people, this is the only story they may have ever heard about the issue, apart from perhaps reading in a trashy tabloid at their hair salon about a few Hollywood celebrities who have had a child via surrogate. To be honest, before my own journey, I generally thought of surrogacy as something that only celebrities did. However, almost every time I tell our story, it generates an entirely different reaction, with people expressing shock and dismay over the challenges

---

15. In July 2014, an internationally publicized incident occurred in which a Thai woman, Pattaramon Janbua, who had been hired as a surrogate for an Australian couple, sought to raise money for her critically ill surrogate son. The baby had been in her care since she gave birth in December 2013; biological parents David John Farnell and Wenyu Wendy Li had left Thailand two months later with baby Gammy's twin sister Pipah.

that we were facing. I have also realized through speaking out on this issue that people are often afraid of the unknown. It is human nature for us to trust and want to protect that which we know and understand, and this is why change is so difficult for a lot of people to accept and ultimately adapt to. Stories assist to break through the invisible barrier that exists, as people tend to learn to adapt to a new idea or way of doing something when they can relate to a story or another person's experience.

We had decided we wanted to move back to Australia before the girls reached school age, so that we could be closer to our family. This was something that would not be possible for our children unless we were able to successfully navigate the legal issues we were facing. Regardless, Australian citizenship was also something I wanted my girls to have because I believe it was their right as the children of two Australians, so I was determined to fight, if needed, to make that happen. As it happened, we found that people were very interested in our story, and we were approached by the Australian Broadcasting Corporation about doing a story on our situation.

We were in the middle of the legal proceedings for our parental rights case and our lawyer was hesitant about us agreeing to do the story because he was worried that doing so could generate an unfavorable decision. I felt strongly that our story needed to be told, purely for the purpose of shedding light on such an important issue, that was largely being ignored. I also felt that if the judge was going to make a ruling based on the fact that we had chosen to speak truthfully about our situation and the issues that exist for families in similar situations, then we have an even bigger problem with our legal system. So, we decided to do the story which aired on the ABC on October 22, 2017.

Sometime after the ABC story, I became involved with Surrogacy Australia and was eventually appointed to the Board as a non-executive director. The work that the organization does is incredibly important because it provides information, resources, and support for intended parents and surrogates in Australia, as well as advocacy at a state and federal level for better laws. The organization aims to influence change to legislation to protect surrogates, intended parents and children in a process which requires careful planning and appropriate legal protections for all parties who are involved in the process, most importantly the child.

The resources and support that Surrogacy Australia provides are typically provided by surrogacy agencies in countries such as the U.S.. However, because commercial surrogacy is not permitted in Australia, there are no surrogacy agencies to provide the resources and support there. Like most charitable organizations though, funds are desperately needed to continue this work and we have a long and tough road ahead before we achieve adequate changes in the law, so that surrogacy might become a realistic possibility for more families in the future.

In January 2018, we obtained Australian citizenship for the girls and an order from the court, in respect to our parental rights case. However, while I would like to tell you the outcome of our application, the judge imposed an order to protect the identity of the children and the surrogate and so I am unable to do so. Our experience with the legal system in Australia though was not the last time that we would encounter issues related to the surrogacy.

In 2019, we decided to move to London for a work opportunity. I hold British citizenship, as my family are from the U.K. and Dave was eligible for a U.K. ancestry visa, as his grandfather was British. I could have applied for a visa for the girls as a result of my citizenship, but it was an easier and quicker process to apply for their visas as part of Dave's application, so we decided on that pathway instead. What we had not anticipated was that the issue of the girls' birth via surrogacy could arise and once again become an issue.

We had assumed that the applications would be fairly straightforward, but as months passed without a decision and with our departure date fast approaching, we had no option but to engage legal counsel in the U.K. to assist. What we quickly discovered though, was that the issue of surrogacy is extremely complex in the U.K. too, and after obtaining a legal opinion from four different firms who provided four different answers, we had no idea whether we were even going to be able to make it to the U.K. In the U.K., surrogacy is legal, but if you make a surrogacy agreement, it cannot be enforced by law. The surrogate will be the child's legal parent at birth and if they are married or in a civil partnership, their spouse or civil partner will be the child's second parent at birth, unless they did not give their permission. Legal parenthood can be transferred by a parental order or adoption after the child is born.

The situation is a lot more complex when it comes to overseas arrangements though, so in our case, what we were unable to determine with any certainty, was whether the court order in Texas granting us parental rights would be valid in the U.K. The legal opinions we obtained were mixed and one of the lawyers we consulted with felt that we would be unable to obtain visas for the girls under either my citizenship or Dave's ancestry application, without first obtaining a separate U.K. parental order. To further complicate things, to obtain a U.K. parental order, the surrogate must consent to the application, or if there is a dispute, the court will make a determination based on what it considers is in the best interests of the child.

Having to go through another legal proceeding was the last thing we wanted to have to do, but needing to involve our surrogate after everything that had happened, was something that was absolutely out of the question as far as I was concerned. I still hadn't healed from the trauma I had experienced because of our surrogate and the thought of ever having to see or speak to her again made me feel physically ill. I just couldn't do it, so we had no choice but to wait and hope for the best.

The weeks, then days leading up to our move were incredibly stressful and there were many tears. Finally, three days before our house was to be packed up by the removal company, the passports were returned to us with the visas inside. I could finally breathe a sigh of relief. We were on our way to a new adventure! The whole experience made me realize though, just how complex the issue of surrogacy is on a global scale, as the laws from one country to the next vary widely. Just when you think the nightmare is over, it can arise again in unexpected ways. For a family who are global, this is always going to be something we have to consider whenever we are travelling, and neither Dave or I will ever be able to blindly consider a job offer in another part of the world, without first asking the questions, "Will the surrogacy be an issue?" and more importantly, "Will our parentage be recognized by this country?" Thinking about it causes me anxiety because we went through so much to create our family.

It feels so incredibly unfair that we are constantly faced with these types of concerns. At the end of the day though, we have our wonderful daughters, and they are without doubt my greatest accomplishment. They are my heart, my soul and my life, and there isn't a day that goes by that I don't feel incredibly grateful and blessed to be able to call myself their mother. So, whatever else might happen and whatever additional challenges we might face in the future, as we continue to navigate these issues in different parts of the world and in different aspects of our life, we are in it together and that thought gives me tremendous power and strength.

Moving On

I am so proud of our little family and how far we have come. We live a perfectly imperfect life that is full of love, adventure and fun and I wouldn't want it any other way. Savannah and Adaline are healthy, happy little girls. I am raising them to be kind humans and I am trying to lead my life as an example for them to follow because it is extremely important to me that they will grow up understanding how blessed and privileged they are and therefore it is imperative that they too should find their own way to give back to others. Right now though, that means donating some of their pocket money, or helping me to hand out money or food to the homeless, but my hope is that this will ultimately set the tone for their own lives as they get older and that in time, they will each find some way to contribute to society and others less fortunate than themselves. How to be a kind human really was the greatest life lesson that my nana taught me and honestly, I get more joy from the work that I am doing to assist others than I do from any of my other professional roles.

Being a parent is not for everyone and that is absolutely fine. But for Dave and me, it is something we both wanted so desperately and we are beyond thrilled to call Savannah and Adaline our children. They fill us with absolute joy. Don't get me wrong, there are daily challenges, and it is hard work, but worth it! I didn't know that this type of pure, unconditional love was possible, until I became their mother. As we were going through the surrogacy journey there were some people who would make completely insensitive comments like, "How will you bond with the babies if you are not carrying them?" and "When does the mother have to give the babies to you?" Well, I am here to tell you that I could not love those little girls any more if I tried, and I am fairly certain that they feel the same way about me.

There were times in my life, even before I was married or had even met Dave, when I wasn't sure whether I would ever be blessed with children. I want every person reading this to know that if it is something that your heart truly desires, then there is always a way. I don't believe any person or government has the right to tell a person what they can and cannot do with their own body. We are so fortunate that we are living at a time when science and modern medicine has made things like surrogacy possible for women who are unable to have children themselves and for gay couples as well. I would not have become the person I am today were it not for my journey to become a parent and the lessons that Savannah and Adaline have taught me along the way. I have found my purpose in life because I have been blessed to be their mother.

Our journey to become parents was extremely tough. There are no mincing words here! It was just bloody tough, and even the events that followed were distressing, but at the end of the day no matter what we went through, I could always hold Savannah and Adaline in my arms, and that made whatever challenge we were facing bearable. Through all of the ups, downs, physical and mental pain, heartache, stress and fear, I experienced in my own life all the things I have outlined within this book about the role each of us plays in contributing to the issue of gender equality. I learnt there are many things that we could, and more importantly, should be doing every day to address this issue and improve opportunities for women and minorities in the workplace. I learnt that even when we think that we are supportive of equal opportunity, sometimes we do things that are really not aligned with that goal and when we realize that, it is our obligation to admit to it and try to do better next time.

I realized that workplaces have a very long way to go and there are things that every single workplace can do to better assist women and minorities to succeed. I learnt there absolutely is a better way to live, other than simply pushing through – because ultimately that is a model that can never be sustained for very long. I learnt that all leaders, especially female leaders, must set the tone within their organizations for how women are perceived, valued, and supported and they must all set good examples for other men and women to follow. I learnt that when we actually stand up and ask for help, or take the time we need to heal, grieve and implement some self-care into our lives, we are more productive, more successful, happier and healthier – and amazing things can happen. I learnt that when

I reflect on my life, I want to be known as someone who loved very much, lived to the full, and who definitely did not confuse having a career with having a life – thanks very much Hillary Clinton![16]

I don't have it all figured out by any means. I too am still growing and learning from others as I continue to speak out on this issue, on behalf of all women. There are companies that are doing wonderful things in this space, and I will continue to highlight these companies and showcase these ideas, so that others too may follow, but unless we all commit to making positive steps towards better conditions in the workplace for women and minorities, I fear that we might never achieve true equality. As the mother of two daughters, that is a thought that both terrifies and angers me. I do not want that to be the reality for any little girl alive today. I do not want to have to stand in front of my daughters one day and tell them the truth about the odds they will be up against when they get to the point of entering the workplace themselves.

So, this book is for them, because I am hoping and praying that gender equality will in their lifetimes be something that will simply become the norm, that it no longer needs to be discussed or seen as an issue.

---

16. Hillary Clinton, Howard University Commencement Speech, 1998.

PART 2

Women's health issues in the workplace

- a handbook for a modern world

Women's Health Issues Are a Workplace Issue - Why It Makes Business Sense to Care

As the number of women in the workforce is declining[17], it is more important than ever before to find better ways to support women to stay in the workforce and to succeed at work. It is my strong belief that this requires us to start thinking about the workplace, and more importantly women within the workplace, a little differently.

By recognizing and supporting employee diversity, organizations can create a more equal playing field, which provides employees with a greater ability to succeed at work and that is fundamentally what workplace equality is all about. When employers find better ways to support their employees through the implementation of policies and benefits that are tailored more specifically to individual needs, it gives them greater opportunity to contribute in a more effective and productive way. When employees feel like their employer cares and they receive the tools and support that they need to succeed, they are much more likely to be loyal to an organization and in turn, this typically reduces cost, improves efficiency, and increases profitability.

Most women at some point in their life will suffer from some kind of female health condition such as menstruation issues, endometriosis, fertility issues, pelvic floor disorders, pregnancy loss or menopause-related issues. So many of these health conditions can be debilitating and cause pain, discomfort and a decrease in quality of life, along with various other symptoms. When a woman is experiencing one of these types of health issues it can, and often does, impact every aspect of her life, including her career.

---

17. https://www.cnbc.com/2021/02/08/womens-labor-force-participation-rate-hit-33-year-low-in-january-2021.html; https://www.rand.org/blog/2020/11/women-are-leaving-the-labor-force-in-record-numbers.html; https://www.cnbc.com/2021/10/14/more-than-300000-women-left-the-labor-force-in-september-.html.

But in almost every situation there are things that an organization can do to better support their female population. Numerous studies across the globe demonstrate that it actually makes business sense for organizations to prioritize finding ways to support women. In turn, this works towards the important goal of closing the gender gap. Why is this important? Well, if we can achieve gender equality, gross domestic product globally is estimated to increase by twenty-eight trillion US dollars. Essentially, if we find better ways to support women, we will increase production and contribute more to the economy. It literally makes business sense to care.

In part two of this book, I will provide you with some tools and resources that every single person can use within their own organizations to start discussions about better support, benefits and policies that support women at work. I will arm you with relevant statistics and some of my own research and strategies to support you along the way. I recognize that not every person is going to have the ability to speak out about these issues and that is okay, but I do believe there are big and small things that each of us can do to work towards gender equality.

For some of us it might mean public advocacy. For some, it might mean introducing new benefits at your board or executive team meetings. For some, it might be speaking out against injustice or discrimination occurring within your workplace, and for others, the change might start at home by educating your daughters to speak up for themselves and teaching your sons about how to support the women in their lives and their female co-workers as they enter the workforce.

Whatever your situation, there are things that each of us can be doing each day to support the cause for better workplace gender equality and my hope is that through this book, sharing my story and my ideas for implementing change, I might empower some of you to do the same.

What is Equality?

The definition of equality in the Oxford dictionary starts with the words, "The state of being equal...." but what does that actually mean? It is something I have spent a lot of time thinking about while experiencing various struggles in my life and my career. Ultimately, my search for the answer to that question has been the catalyst for writing this book. I think that most people don't actually know what it means and if people lack an understanding about what equality is, then how can we expect them to appreciate why it is so important in life and in the workplace?

I wanted to test the theory as I was writing this book and what I found is that it is a topic that makes a lot of people feel uncomfortable, even if they are supportive of gender or race equality for example, and when you ask someone to tell you what they think it means, a lot of people stumble and cannot really answer the question. However, the typical answer is something like this, "Everyone being treated the same" or "Everyone being paid the same". These kinds of answers got me thinking that maybe there isn't enough useful information out there to really break down the issue and educate people on what equality is.

I decided to start the second part of the book by diving into this topic to discuss it in more detail. My hope is that by doing so, I can share my insights and thoughts on the issue through my own lived experiences, years of work as an international lawyer, and research – so that you can start thinking about equality in a different way in every area of your life. Like anything, if we have a greater understanding of an issue, it encourages deeper thought, discussion and more effective problem solving. Now, if you will indulge me, I will go ahead and share my thoughts with you.

Diversity and inclusion have become buzz words over recent years. Almost all major companies globally recognize the importance of striving for a diverse workforce that is supportive of its employees – or at least the importance of being seen to do so. Some countries have laws that mandate gender equality in one form or another.

For example, on January 2, 2016, the Brazilian Law on the *Inclusion of Persons with Disabilities*[18] came into effect, which requires all employers to meet a quota of employment of people with disabilities. The quota ranges from two to five percent depending on company size. In Australia, the *Workplace Gender Equality Act 2012* (Cth)[19] requires all employers with one hundred or more employees to report annually on the steps being taken in the workplace to ensure gender equality for both men and women.

In the U.K., menopause in the workplace was a topic of hot debate in 2019, with a number of British MPs pushing for mandated workplace policies to protect women going through menopause. Although we have not heard a lot since, the issue is once again under consideration and focus groups on the U.K. have been asked to report on the issue so that changes to the law can be considered. Currently in the U.K., menopause at work is covered under the *Equality Act 2010*[20] and the *Health and Safety at Work Act 1974*[21] which includes working conditions for those experiencing menopausal symptoms. However, despite these protections, there are few cases where menopause is cited; which is why the law is currently being reviewed and reform is being considered. The Welsh government has also put into place guidance for its workers, advising that all reasonable adjustments should be considered when a health issue may be impacting on a person's ability to carry out their role. This can include changing working location or conditions for a more comfortable working life.

In the U.S., some states now mandate certain gender diversity requirements for boards. For example, in 2018 California introduced board diversity mandates for public companies with their principal executive offices located in California. The law requires any companies that meet these requirements to have at least one woman on its board of directors. Washington state has similar board diversity requirements for public companies which

---

18. (Law no. 13,146/2015) http://planalto.gov.br/ccivil_03/_Ato2015-2018/2015/Lei/L13146.htm

19. http://www8.austlii.edu.au/cgi-bin/viewdb/au/legis/cth/consol_act/wgea2012265/

20. https://www.legislation.gov.uk/ukpga/2010/15/contents

21. https://www.hse.gov.uk/legislation/hswa.htm

was introduced in June 2020. The Washington state law provides that at least twenty-five percent of board members must be women by January 1, 2022 or the company must disclose in its annual proxy statement to shareholders or post on the company's primary website a "board diversity discussion and analysis" that includes information regarding the company's approach to developing and maintaining board diversity. Hawaii, Massachusetts, Michigan, and New Jersey are also currently considering mandatory board diversity legislation that resembles California's gender diversity statute. New York adopted mandatory disclosure requirements in 2020, joining Illinois and Maryland in imposing reporting requirements, which again is aimed at assisting to improve diversity at the board level.

However, despite some countries now having laws which require employers to take positive steps to improve gender diversity in the workplace, unfortunately a lot of companies implement policies to tick the box of compliance and merely pay lip service to diversity and inclusion without ever really taking the time to understand what it means practically for their business and, more importantly, for their employees.

So, what does equality look like in the workplace context, or rather, what should it look like? Well, I think that it is an interesting question and one that we really need to explore if we want to move the needle closer towards achieving gender equality. The aims of equality and diversity are simple: to ensure that everyone has access to the same opportunities and the same, fair treatment. It also means ensuring that people are accepted for their differences. But what exactly does this all mean? I have a few theories that I would like to share with you.

If we went around a room and asked fifty people what workplace equality means to them, I am almost sure that we would end up with fifty different responses. And why? It is because we are all different people. We all have different views and beliefs, and while there are certainly similarities in the lives of one person to the next, no person is the same as another and we all have different responsibilities, pressures, demands and needs in our lives and this includes the workplace as well.

So, if we asked an employee with a physical disability what they believe workplace equality means, they might say something like: "Equality to me would be having my employer provide a workplace where all employees who have physical limitations can access the same areas and facilities as able-bodied employees". If we asked a mother with small children what workplace equality means, she might say something like: "Equality to me would be having an employer allow flexible work times for all employees. This would enable men and women and parents and non-parents the same opportunities to work and prove our abilities on projects without fear of a negative perception of unavailability or the need for flexibility". If we asked a young man what workplace equality means to him, he might say something like: "Employers considering candidates and employees for opportunities without regard to their gender, race etc." And, if we asked an older woman in her sixties what workplace equality means to her, she might say, "An employer who considers and values all employees equally, including younger workers with fresh ideas and older workers with maturity, knowledge and experience".

None of these answers are incorrect, but they are representative of an individual's view of the world and if we fail to recognize that we are all looking at the workplace through our own individual lenses, and the view that we see is colored by our own life experiences, then we fail to understand that in order to have access to the same opportunities, it requires the workplace to better accommodate for the diversity of its people. If we accept that every single person is different, it naturally follows that we all have different experiences at work, and so it should come as no surprise then that a one-size-fits-all approach to the workplace typically doesn't work. The numbers do not lie; what we know without a doubt is that currently women face more barriers and challenges in the workplace than men for many reasons, including the fact that the workplace construct was set up by men for men, and little has changed over the decades since the office environment was born.

Prior to the global pandemic, it was estimated to take at least one hundred years to achieve workplace gender equality. Now, that number is staggering alone – but COVID-19 has had an even greater impact on workplace equality with women being disproportionately impacted. Women are withdrawing from the workforce at alarming rates, with millions of women globally having left the workplace since the pandemic started, and the research is showing us that many do not plan to return. For some, that may be a choice but for many, it has been necessary. The pandemic has caused us to lose decades of the progress that had been made for women and workers at risk, and the gender gap is now estimated to take an additional thirty-six years to close – that's now approximately 135.6 years for women and men to reach parity.

Now I don't know about you, but to me that number is simply unacceptable because it means that my daughters are unlikely to ever see gender equality in their lifetimes and, if you have daughters or granddaughters, it means the same thing for them. We simply must find a way to improve these statistics. We need to start recognizing the roles that women play, both in the workplace context and more generally, and investing time and money into discovering and understanding the unique strengths of women and how best to support them. This is crucial to the workplace gender gap discussion because without this context we are attempting to create a level playing field within the workplace, with players that are entering on unequal footing. It would be like timing two people to complete a puzzle, but one has one arm behind their back while balancing a cup on their head and calling it an equal competition.

By recognizing and supporting employee diversity and their differences, organizations can tailor the workplace environment to create a truly equal playing field which, in turn, provides employees with a greater ability to succeed at work – and that is fundamentally what workplace equality is all about.

An organization's people are its most important asset, and they also represent one of its largest investments. Like most investments, how much time you spend researching, understanding, and nurturing the investment often determines the return. Almost every company around the world has similar goals – to have productive employees and to be profitable. To get the very best out of people, it is imperative that organizations invest the time to understand the diversity of their workforce. Just as companies invest resources in understanding their customers, so too should they when it comes to their employees. Some employees are parents, some are carers, some have disabilities, and some have health issues that they are trying to manage while seeking to perform their best at work. Our experiences at work are therefore all very different and so it follows that the support and resources that we need to succeed will be different as well. Yet despite this, most organizations still apply a one-size-fits-all approach to workplace conditions, policies and benefits and they fail to invest the time and resources in building workplaces that fit the needs of their employees to assist them to achieve their best for the organization.

I think that there are smarter ways that most organizations can invest in their people and there are improvements that every single employer can make to better support their employees at work. Not only do I think this is crucial to a successful diversity and inclusion strategy, and essential if we are going to reach gender parity in the workplace, but I also strongly believe it is every employer's obligation to prioritize employee health and wellness. COVID-19 has demonstrated to us all the impact that isolation and loneliness can have on every one of us, and to a woman who suffers a health condition or pregnancy loss in silence, they are particularly vulnerable to feelings of isolation, anxiety and depression without appropriate resources and support.

There is no doubt in my mind that the number of people suffering from some form of mental health issue has risen since the start of the pandemic. After all, how could they not? As scientist Matthew Lieberman details in his book *Social*[22], our need to connect with other people is even more fundamental than some of our other basic needs, such as food. Research conducted by Lieberman shows that our brains react to social pain and pleasure in much the same way as they do to physical pain and pleasure. Relevant to recent events globally, the data suggests we are profoundly shaped by our social environment and we suffer greatly when our social bonds are threatened or severed. COVID-19 has been the global experiment we

---

22. https://www.penguinrandomhouse.com/books/212681/social-by-matthew-d-lieberman/

never wanted; one that has demonstrated to us just how much we each rely on and need the support of one another.

Some of my loved ones suffer from depression, and I have watched from afar, broken-hearted, as they have struggled over the last two years. Being restricted from seeing them due to lockdowns and closed international borders, there is little I have been able to do. In my legal work, I have also seen a significant rise in the number of employee mental health cases that have come across my desk since the pandemic started. Every week I see more and more employees who are struggling with not just the physical aspects of COVID-19 as they try to navigate the inability to travel, visit customers and work collaboratively with their teams in-person – but many are also juggling family responsibilities with school closures occurring on and off in almost every country around the world.

My own experiences both personally and professionally have left me with a sense of certainty about just how important it is for employers to recognize the role that each and every leader and employee plays in managing and prioritizing mental health. While we are not all doctors, we need to develop a better understanding of the ways that every one of us can better support our employees at work, especially as the lines between work and personal life have become so blurred and, in many cases, are now non-existent.

Stress has a more significant impact on our bodies than most of us actually realize. I can tell you from first-hand experience just how important having a supportive workplace is to a person suffering from any kind of health issue and without a doubt, stress itself can cause a range of physical impacts. Everything from headaches, migraines, anxiety, eating disorders, angry outbursts, insomnia, fatigue, bowel problems, depression and more. Stress can also cause or exacerbate more serious health problems, including endometriosis and fertility issues.

One of the things that a doctor often tells a patient struggling to conceive is that they just need to relax and try not to stress. Easy said. Hard to do. When you are desperately wanting to start a family, you are often in a state of almost constant stress and anxiety, thinking of little else. We have all heard those stories of couples who struggle to have a child for years and years, finally adopting only to end up pregnant once they have moved on and stopped focusing on getting pregnant. Stress can disable the body's immune system, making it unable to function properly and therefore make us more susceptible to illness. Unfortunately, it also tends to become a vicious cycle. The more we stress, the more unwell we become. The more unwell we become, the more stressed we are that our body is limiting our ability to perform work and other everyday functions and so on it goes in circles. Sometimes people even experience symptoms of stress without actually realizing that stress is the cause of the underlying issue. This happened to me.

About six months after I started writing this book, I began to experience some health issues. I didn't recognize that they might be related to the fact that I was writing about some really painful experiences but as I finished part one of the book and the symptoms started to subside, I realized it probably wasn't a coincidence.

One evening I was out at a friend's birthday dinner and another friend who I had not seen for some time was also there. We got talking and she told me that her sister had recently passed away suddenly. She told that her sister was in her early thirties with a young child and because of this, she had not gone to the doctor when she first started experiencing symptoms. My friend's sister had been experiencing similar symptoms to what I was, and this poor woman ended up with stage four cancer and passing away three months after she was diagnosed. It frightened me enough that I went home and promised my husband that I would make an appointment the following Monday to see a specialist.

I kept my word and called a gastroenterologist. I was told they had about a three-month wait list but when they asked me the problem and I detailed my symptoms, they told me I'd better come in right away. That frightened me, but in I went. After multiple tests and further symptoms developing that were now more akin to those I had always experienced as a result of my endometriosis, I started to realize it was all probably related and ultimately, the gastroenterologist reached the same conclusion. I was five months down the track and no closer to relief. I hadn't really felt symptoms associated with endometriosis since my last surgery in 2019. Back then, my symptoms had presented differently as well, which is why endo had not entered my mind, however, it soon became clear to me what was happening inside my body. I was frustrated with my body and my mind, but I realized something with some certainty – just how significant a role stress plays and the impact it can have on a person's health.

Thankfully, as I progressed through the book and was able to put the part about my story to bed, my health did start to improve, and I was able to continue on. However, it set me back and ultimately caused a delay in finishing the book and I think that it is also important to point that out for another reason. That is to tell you that self-improvement is an everlasting journey. There is no magic pill. Everyone has ups and downs. Everyone has good days and bad days. Everyone experiences joy and sadness, and everyone has successes and failures. The important thing is to realize that, and on those days that are bad, full of sadness or disappointments, to get back up and try to do better tomorrow. That is ultimately all any of us can expect of ourselves or of others. Unfortunately, though, what so many of us do is apply a standard to ourselves and others that fails to account for our human experiences.

We cannot ignore the fact that there is often a stigma attached to absence or leave. It can be unconscious, but unfortunately it is significant enough that almost one-third of U.S. workers are concerned about taking a leave of absence[23]. In some countries such as Australia, Britain and parts of Europe, where culturally leave is more accepted as a normal occurrence, employees will regularly take extended periods to vacation, rest and recuperate. An email 'out of office' is also not uncommon there. Compare this to the U.S or China however, and the opposite is typically true. I have heard company leaders issue directives against email notifications that advise clients of unavailability for fear of any negative perception of reliability attached to an 'out of office' email. This type of directive sends a clear message that this is an area of vulnerability that demonstrates weakness, a hole or gap in what we want others to believe is a perfect system. This is the type of thinking

23. The Hartford Financial Services Group, Inc.'s 2021 Future of Benefits Study: https://www.thehartford.com/employee-benefits/employ-ers/insights/future-of-benefits-2021

that leaves no room for humanity or the realities of life. 'We are all just human', is not a statement that fits well within this type of institution and there is certainly no sign of advocacy for 'bring your whole self to work' type policies (whatever they actually mean!).

When it comes to women, who may need to take time off work or have flexibility to deal with health issues, fertility challenges, medical appointments due to pregnancy or for childcare responsibilities for example, the situation is even worse and still today we know that women are often subjected to discriminatory and unfair treatment as a result. Over the years, I have seen countless examples of women saying, "I am going through X, and I need some time to do Y", who are then labelled as "uncommitted", "not up to the task" or "lacking leadership qualities" when the time comes to consider her for a promotion or new work opportunity. In situations like this, when I have asked for examples, many times I have been told that someone has made the decision that the individual is just not the right fit or that she doesn't have what is needed for the role, but tangible or measurable examples to explain the decision cannot be provided.

As the American business magnate, investor and philanthropist Warren Buffet said, "It takes 20 years to build a reputation and five minutes to ruin it. If you think about that, you'll do things differently." Buffet was of course talking about having integrity in business, but I believe that this is also the reason why many people are fearful of asking their employer for flexibility and leave when needed. Reputation internally is also just as important as your external reputation in the market, because if you are respected within your organization, you are more likely to be supported. When life happens and you do need to take time away from work, a company that respects and supports you will find ways to manage your clients and the message to the marketplace when you are not available.

As I was writing this book, I put a call out for other women to tell me their stories. Many women came forward to share their experiences and struggles in the workplace and I am incredibly grateful to those women for trusting me enough to do so, especially because many of their stories involve extremely painful experiences. What became evident though, was that there was a recurring theme throughout many of their stories. That is, time and again women would need to take time away from their jobs for reasons related to personal health or family, and they would return to find that their role had been impacted as a result. Someone else was now in the role and they were expected to simply step aside gracefully.

In some cases, they were never able to return at all and were effectively pushed out of the organization. And why? Well, we will never know the actual reasons and what discussions occurred behind closed doors in each situation, but what we do know is that these are the types of experiences that women have every day around the world, because taking time away from work or asking for flexibility are often not things that are associated with the ideal model employee. They don't go hand-in-hand with our idea of hard work, dedication and commitment – all of the attributes that we have come to value in a 'good employee', and this is exactly why we continue to push through and show up when we are physically or mentally unwell, even when it is to our own detriment. I have fallen into this trap myself many times.

In my view, to achieve workplace gender equality, we need to start to look at our ideas around what it means to be a good employee. This requires employers to open their minds to different ways of thinking about the workplace and effective ways to work. It also requires employers to look at the value they place on certain attributes in their employees and how they measure success and strong performance, and this requires a mindset shift.

If we know that diverse teams outperform regular teams, then it should follow that we recognize that our teams should not all look the same. Rather, they should be made up of team members from different ethnic backgrounds. They should include men and women. There should be heterosexual members and members of the LGBTIQ+ community. There should be non-disabled employees and employees with disabilities and if our teams are truly diverse then we should stop expecting every person in that team to perform based on a standard, one-size-fits-all approach to workplace policies and practices. Essentially, for diverse teams to thrive, we need diversity in approach and what this actually looks like will depend on the nature of the workplace, the employee's position and the requirements for the role.

I believe our idea of what equality is needs some work, because there is a general perception that if we put everyone in the ring, then they all have a chance to succeed and that's equality. That is a skewed idea that fundamentally lacks consideration for the environment around us and it assumes we are therefore all entering the ring on an equal playing field, with an equal chance of success. As we know though, that is far from the reality, because women are often already at a disadvantage for many reasons. We are at a disadvantage because women often carry more of the childcare and home life responsibilities in a family. Women suffer more health issues than men and women see fewer faces similar to their own at the top of organizations, which has both psychological effects and also very real, tangible impacts when decisions are made within organizations.

To reach a state where women have more equal opportunities to succeed at work, we have to consider better ways to support women in their career journeys. The research shows us there is a direct link between productivity and wellness, and when you find ways to really support your employees, they in turn will support the organization through increased productivity, less turnover and reduced business cost such as recruitment and health care costs. As highlighted throughout **What Innovative Companies Around the World Are Doing to Tackle This Issue**, those organizations that have worked this out are seeing significant cost savings and benefits.

We all have a role to play to achieve workplace equality. If we want to see change in workplaces and more supportive employers, then we too each need to play our part. We need to work hard whenever we are able, and, where possible, we need to actively come up with solutions rather than just approaching our employers with problems. Law makers also have a role to play in this issue, but the reality is that laws often take far too long to change, and we are stuck with a legal framework that can be in place for decades or, in some cases, even centuries. Just another reason why we need more women in top positions within governments to effect change around issues impacting women. I, for one, am pretty sure that we would get things done a lot faster if there were more of us sitting within governments.

Female-Only Health Issues and the Impact at the Office

Women and men are genetically and biologically different – that's a fact. Research conducted in 2017 revealed that there are actually 6,500 genes that are different in men and women[24]. Other studies have showed identical genes can work differently in men and women. One such study conducted by Stanford University suggested the research could help explain why there are discrepancies in health and disease between men and women that scientists don't fully understand. However, quite simply because we have different body parts and our bodies function differently in some ways, there are a large number of health issues that are unique to women.

While women are affected by many of the same health conditions as men, the diseases affect them differently and often women are at higher risk. There are also many gender-specific diseases and health conditions that only affect women. Major risks to women's health include cardiovascular disease, cancer, osteoporosis, and depression. Women are more likely to be diagnosed with stress and depression than men. Osteoarthritis, a disease that causes joint tissue to break down over time causing pain and stiffness in hand, knee, hips, neck, and lower back joints, affects more women than men. It is also the leading cause of disability in the United States[25].

Depression and major depressive disorder (MDD) are more prevalent among women compared to men, and the differences are most prominent during the reproductive years. Genes, hormones, and stress can all contribute to these conditions. When hormones change, brain chemistry also changes, which is why some women experience depression after having a baby and during or after

24. https://www.dailymail.co.uk/sciencetech/article-4475252/There-6-500-genetic-differences-men-women.html

25. https://www.drugwatch.com/health/arthritis/osteoarthritis/

menopause. Periods of hormonal variability, such as the luteal phase of the menstrual cycle, the postpartum period, and the menopausal transition, represent times when a substantial subset of women experience mood disturbances. Normal shifts in endogenous reproductive hormone levels can contribute to pathological mood episodes in women, and one can hypothesize that MDD might in fact represent a highly heterogeneous disorder that can be better characterized among subsets of women in comparison to men[26]. The female reproductive hormones can also impact mood at each stage of the reproductive health life cycle.

Women are at higher risk for metabolic syndrome, a condition that increases the risk of heart disease, stroke, and diabetes. It includes high blood pressure, high blood sugar, excess body fat around the waist, and abnormal cholesterol levels. More women suffer from lupus, which is an autoimmune disease, than men. Cardiovascular disease is the number one killer of women, causing one in three deaths each year. That's approximately one woman every minute! African American women are disproportionately affected by heart disease, leading the death rate regardless of age and Hispanic women are likely to develop heart disease ten years earlier than non-Hispanics. Approximately forty-two percent of women who have a heart attack die within a year compared to twenty-four percent of men. Lung cancer is the leading type of cancer that causes death in women, with breast cancer the second most likely.

Women are more susceptible to osteoporosis in later life than men. Women aged fifty years or older have a four times higher rate of osteoporosis and a two times higher rate of osteopenia compared with men. This is due to the hormone changes that happen during menopause, which impacts bone density. Eighty-five percent of the total number of people diagnosed with anorexia nervosa or bulimia nervosa are women. People with these eating disorders can experience mental health problems, heart problems, blood problems kidney problems, intestine problems, hormone problems and problems with their skin, hair, muscles, joints, and bones.

---

26. https://www.ncbi.nlm.nih.gov/pmc/articles/PMC4096821/

Women also experience unique female-only health issues and conditions, from pregnancy and menopause to gynecological conditions, such as uterine fibroids and pelvic floor disorders as well as many others including the following:

- **menstruation and menstrual irregularities**
- **urinary tract health issues**, including such disorders as bacterial vaginosis, vaginitis, uterine fibroids, and vulvodynia
- **Pregnancy issues** include pre-pregnancy care and prenatal care, pregnancy loss (miscarriage and stillbirth), preterm labor and premature birth, sudden infant death syndrome (SIDS), breastfeeding, and birth defects
- **Disorders related to infertility** include uterine fibroids, polycystic ovary syndrome, endometriosis, and primary ovarian insufficiency
- **Menopause** and various health issues and associated symptoms
- **Other disorders and conditions** that affect only women include Turner syndrome, Rett syndrome, and ovarian and cervical cancers.

Many of these female-only health conditions can cause significant side-effects, which themselves can lead to other issues in a chain reaction. For example, blood loss related to various uterine issues can lead to anaemia, exhaustion, extreme fatigue and difficulty concentrating. For a professional woman who feels the pressure to keep performing, this may lead her to resort to medications or excessive caffeine consumption, which in turn have side effects such as kidney problems and sleep disorders.

Similarly, headaches and migraines, back pain, faintness or nausea have ongoing effects on the woman's lifestyle and health and the medications necessary to allow her to lead a relatively normal life and continue working effectively may have serious side effects. These may include higher risk of heart attacks, strokes, blood clots, organ damage, increased risk of cancer and birth defects in unborn children.

In addition to the physical symptoms, side-effects and risks associated with medications for treatment, it is also important to recognize that some female health problems can have a significant emotional impact and, in some cases, also cause mental health issues that can be particularly severe shortly after diagnosis and following a long history of experience with a disease or disorder. For example, the psychological impact on a woman who experiences ongoing fertility issues can be severe and can result in significant additional conditions such as depression, anxiety and panic attacks.

It therefore comes as no surprise to me to learn that women are seventy percent more likely to experience severe clinical depression than men. Postpartum depression is a common form of depression in women, but depression can be triggered by many factors and at any age. As a woman who experienced many of the health issues identified above, I can relate to this. Of course, at the time I did not realize I was depressed or that I had any additional health issues that were triggered by the other conditions that my body was suffering, but the reality is that they were.

There was no greater example of this in motion for me than shortly after I had a hysterectomy and we were going through the process of (a) coming to terms with the fact that I would no longer physically be able to get pregnant; (b) what that meant was that I was actually not going to be able to give birth to my own child; (c) trying to manage the change in my body, the healing that my body needed to do and the hormonal changes that I was experiencing; and (d) trying to manage the surrogacy process that we had just embarked on. I was trying to do all of these things at once and so it should not have come as any surprise when a mere few months after having the hysterectomy, I was once again back in my gynecologist's office complaining of severe back pain and begging her to help me. After an examination and some tests, we determined that the endometriosis had returned spreading to different parts of my body this time.

So, back into hospital for my tenth surgery I went. It was actually that surgery that changed my life, because as I was lying in the hospital bed going through the pre-surgery steps before I was wheeled into the operating theatre, I made a promise to myself. I told myself that day that I would make changes in my life. I would stop pushing myself to inhuman levels. I would start being kinder to myself and treating myself better than I had been for all this time.

I am not going to tell you I woke up after the surgery and everything in my life was magically fixed. That is definitely not what happened. In fact, it was far from the case and for a while I did a poor job of taking care of myself. I made less than optimal choices by continuing to push through and I kept going at times when I really needed to take time to rest and heal. There were still many days when I literally had nothing left to give; yet I would push on, sometimes crying at night out of sheer exhaustion. I am not ashamed of that. It is simply part of my story and I want to tell you the truth so that hopefully you will not make the same mistakes that I did, or at least not as many! What I can tell you though is that I did start making small steps in the right direction and eventually I got myself to a much better place. You know what else? Surprise, surprise! Once I became a bit healthier, I was a LOT happier, and my work performance improved too! So, by taking better care of myself I ended up being more successful and, actually increasing my productivity and profitability.

Don't get me wrong, I have always been a hard worker and I have never failed to achieve my financial targets, but once I started to shift things in my life in a more positive direction and improve my own health and priorities by creating a lot more balance in my life, not only did I see noticeable improvements, but those around me benefited as well, including my employer. Now, if that isn't a great advertisement for self-improvement and health and wellness, then I don't know what is.

Before I get to what I actually did to improve my life and the steps I took along that journey, I have a lot more to tell you. During the ten months that I lived in London, I was working nights, raising my daughters largely on my own as my husband was living in Los Angeles, and there was little time for sleep, let alone any self-care. During the first year of the COVID-19 pandemic, like many people I was juggling my children and an influx of work, with clients desperately trying to scramble to keep up with a world that had changed overnight and workplaces that had to immediately adapt.

I worked many long days through that period, as well as right through many nights. In both cases, I struggled, and my health suffered significantly. In London, I ended up with pneumonia and had to be 'rescued' by my poor brother Ben, who flew from Australia to help me with the twins. During the pandemic I started to have symptoms that I was almost certain meant that I was having a heart attack. In fact, I was so sure that something serious was wrong with me that my doctor decided to run every test he could possibly think of to ensure there was actually nothing wrong with my heart.

I could be sitting at my desk drafting, when I would suddenly experience shooting pains down one arm and through the left side of my chest. Or at night, I would just lie down in bed to drift off to sleep and I would experience horrible pain in my chest and tingling in my arms and legs. At the end of a month of testing, scans, blood tests and appointments, all which showed that there was nothing in fact wrong at all with my heart, my doctor finally said to me, "Naomi, have you thought that maybe this is anxiety. I mean, come on. You realize that your workload is not normal, right?" My immediate reaction was to dismiss that idea as crazy. I had experienced anxiety when I was about nineteen years old, and it was nothing at all like this.

Another thing I am not proud of is that I had been having these terrible symptoms for over two months – pain in my arm, chest and tingling down my arms and legs - before I finally relented to my husband Dave's demands that I go to see the doctor. And why did I not go? Well, again, same old story. I simply just didn't have time. My clients needed me desperately throughout the pandemic, and when I wasn't working, I had to devote every minute that I had to being present for my children.

I felt guilty enough about the amount that I was working, and I couldn't afford to take any more of my time away from them. So, once again I pressed on. I want to stress that ANYONE who is experiencing any of the types of symptoms that you should absolutely NEVER wait as long as I did to seek treatment. People die every day from heart disease and heart attack, and it can happen so quickly. Thankfully, in my case I was fine, and it wasn't my heart at all, but you simply never know. It is just not worth the risk of waiting to seek help.

I have since discovered that heart attack is something that actually kills more women than men. Interestingly, while men have more heart attacks than women, women suffer higher heart attack deaths compared to men. Could this be another example of women pushing through, not wanting to (or possibly having the time to) raise issues of personal illness until it is all too late, while men are more likely to seek help at earlier signs of something being wrong? I am not a doctor and I don't know the answer to that question with any certainly, but what I do know is that experts in the area do believe that one of the reasons for this is that women who suffer a heart attack often have more untreated risk factors such as diabetes or high blood pressure and it is sometimes because women will put their families (and others generally – often also including their employers!) first and don't take care of themselves. Now *that* I can definitely accept as true and most certainly can relate to. Nonetheless, it is an interesting statistic and one that deserves some thought and reflection.

REPRODUCTIVE HEALTH

The reproductive cycle affects many stages of a woman's life from adolescence right through to old age. There are five reproductive stages in a woman's reproductive life cycle. These include the premenarchal (before the first menstrual period) stage; the reproductive, premenopausal stage; the early menopausal transition stage; the late menopausal transition stage; and finally, menopause. Each stage can present different health challenges for a woman.

At approximately eight years of age, girls begin to product estrogen. Girls start menstruating between the ages of ten and fifteen. The average age is twelve, but it varies from person to person and between countries, as it is believed that in addition to genes, environment, climate and diet may also have an impact. A woman's reproductive period lasts between the time of first menstruation (following puberty) through to approximately five to ten years before menopause. A woman's best reproductive years are generally in her twenties. A growing number of couples are experiencing infertility, with approximately one in six now seeking treatment. Fertility naturally declines as a woman ages, which makes it harder to conceive and having children later in life poses greater risk for pregnancy complications. Age-related infertility is becoming more common because many women are waiting until their thirties to start trying to have a family.

Even though women today are healthier and there is more of a focus on health and wellness globally, because we have a better understanding of the importance of this, improved health unfortunately does not offset the natural age-related decline in fertility. To put it into context, a healthy thirty-year-old woman has a twenty percent chance of getting pregnant in any month. By age forty, a woman's chance of getting pregnant is less than five percent per month. Egg quality also significantly declines as a woman ages. You can therefore imagine just how difficult it is for women with fertility or other health issues to get pregnant. It really is a miracle whenever any woman gets pregnant – health issues or not!

Many women are hesitant to share their infertility struggles for fear that it will impact negatively upon their careers. According to researched conducted by Fertility Network UK[27] in 2016, approximately fifty percent of women undergoing fertility treatments do not disclose it to their employers because of a belief that their employer would not take them seriously and over forty percent due to the concerns about negative impacts on their career.

Interestingly, in an interview that was reported in *The Guardian* in March 2021[28] Shanna Swan, a professor of environmental medicine and public health at the Icahn School of Medicine at Mount Sinai (formerly the Mount Sinai School of Medicine), said that chemicals in plastics are causing our fertility to decline, and it is her belief that by 2045 "most couples" may have to use assisted reproduction. A scary thought indeed, but one the demonstrates the extent of the issue and its impact on the workforce.

Another unseen consequence of fertility issues and the inevitable treatments that so many women are forced to undergo, is the impact on the gender pay gap. As men advance in their careers

---

27. https://fertilitynetworkuk.org/wp-content/uploads/2016/10/SURVEY-RESULTS-Impact-of-Fertility-Problems.pdf

28. https://www.theguardian.com/society/2021/mar/28/shanna-swan-fertility-reproduction-count-down?fbclid=IwAR0lJBlBaR-3bJ2aqwueEOch5qD5fkOuu84qAgbuoHr_lHYAzJ9t-FFxne9E

and are able to save income towards major purchases, women are now losing billions of dollars of earnings to invest in their futures through fertility treatments such as egg freezing. The cost of fertility treatments like this can be anywhere from $20,000 to $60,000 with most medical insurance plans not covering these types of treatments. As Tammy Sun so eloquently put it in her Fortune article in April 2021: "**'Equal pay' won't be truly equal until fertility care is covered** Tammy says, "As we work for gender pay equity, we should also be thinking about how to close the gap by making fertility care accessible and affordable to all. The workplace is a logical first step[29]".

MENSTRUAL IRREGULARITIES AND ASSOCIATED CONDITIONS

The menstrual cycle is a series of changes that occur to a woman's ovaries, uterus, vagina, and breasts, on average every twenty-eight days, although the duration of a cycle can vary. The average menstrual period lasts about five to seven days.

Menstrual cycle disorders are common and can include:

- Heavy menstrual bleeding: one in five women suffer from heavy menstrual bleeding. Blood loss during a normal menstrual period is about five tablespoons, but some women experience bleeding up to twenty-five times this amount each month. It can be so debilitating for some women that they cannot perform everyday functions. It can cause extreme exhaustion, migraines, anemia, and various other associated health conditions.
- Severe menstrual cramps (dysmenorrhea): At some point in their lives, most women will experience painful cramps during a period. Cramps that are especially painful are called dysmenorrhea and can require medical intervention, as other symptoms such as diarrhea, faintness and low blood pressure can also follow.

29. https://fortune-com.cdn.ampproject.org/c/s/fortune.com/2021/04/05/fertility-care-benefits-ivf-egg-freezing-equal-pay-act/amp/

- Premenstrual syndrome (PMS): PMS appears to be caused by rising and falling levels of the hormones estrogen and progesterone, which may influence brain chemicals, including serotonin. PMS is a combination of symptoms that over ninety percent of woman say that they experience about a week or two before their period. There are more than 150 documented symptoms of PMS including bloating, headaches, mood swings, tender breasts, food cravings, fatigue, irritability, and depression. Approximately thirty to forty percent of women experience symptoms so severe that it causes a disruption to their everyday life. Symptoms of PMS may increase in severity following each pregnancy and may worsen with age until menopause. There are currently no specific diagnostic tests for PMS.
- Premenstrual Dysphoric Disorder (PMDD): PMDD is a severe form of premenstrual syndrome that includes physical and behavioral symptoms including extreme mood swings, extreme sadness, feelings of hopelessness, irritability and anger, as well as breast tenderness and bloating. There are currently no specific diagnostic tests for PMDD. Medication or surgery may be required to treat PMDD.

ENDOMETRIOSIS

Endometriosis is a disease in which the endometrium (the tissue that lines the inside of the uterus or womb) is present outside of the uterus. Endometriosis most commonly occurs in the lower abdomen or pelvis, but it may surprise you to learn that it can actually appear anywhere in the body. There are cases of women who have had endometriosis in the bowel, bladder, stomach, joints, lungs and even the brain. Symptoms can include lower abdominal pain, lower back pain, pain with menstrual periods, pain with sexual intercourse, extreme fatigue, nausea, and difficulty getting pregnant. For the one in ten women globally (approximately 200 million women) who suffer with endometriosis, it can be debilitating. Unfortunately, I am one of those women, and I know too well the significant impact that it can have on your quality of life, not to mention the time and money spent on lost days of work and medical costs associated with seeking a diagnosis and then ongoing treatment. On average, the cost of endometriosis to women suffering from the disease is approximately $30,000 a year[30].

Currently, surgery (a laparoscopy) is the only way to make a formal diagnosis of endometriosis. This is where a small camera is inserted into the pelvic/abdominal cavity to investigate the presence of endometriosis lesions. Because there is no good noninvasive test for endometriosis, there is often a significant delay in diagnosis. On average it can take six-and-a-half years for a woman to be diagnosed with endometriosis because most endometriosis can only be diagnosed through surgery, which is always a last resort. Globally, there remains little funding for endometriosis research, and it is still a largely misunderstood disease. Current statistics show sixty-four percent of women aged sixteen to twenty-four have never heard of endometriosis and eighty percent would put off going to the doctor even if they were experiencing symptoms.

It is currently estimated that at least eleven percent of women in the U.S. and Australia, ten percent of women in the U.K. and about one in ten or ten percent of all women globally suffer from endometriosis. However, the figures could be even higher because of the delay in the average diagnosis. Endometriosis is also often misdiagnosed. Although I was diagnosed at a fairly young age of twenty-two, I too have experienced the issues surrounding diagnosis since. I have lost count of how many laparoscopies I have had for my endometriosis, but my body certainly shows the little scars at various points of my pelvis to prove it. On at least three occasions though, my gynecologist was not able to see any signs of endometriosis on the scans. It was only a result of knowing my history that led my doctor to proceed to a surgery each time.

My last endometriosis surgery was in September 2019, and it was my most complicated surgery, as the endometriosis had spread

---

30. https://www.endometriosisaustralia.org/; https://theconversation.com/endometriosis-costs-women-and-society-30-000-a-year-for-every-sufferer-124975

into my bowel and urinary tract. In the weeks leading up to that surgery, I was experiencing pain in my lower back so severe that there were days when I could not stand up and it caused almost a hallucinatory state. Pain medications offered little relief. My doctor scheduled me for surgery, but the pain became so unbearable that I was forced to rush to the emergency department one day and the surgery had to be performed that afternoon.

The result was that I ended up with severe nerve damage because of the extent to which the endometriosis had spread. The pain that followed as a result of the nerve damage was so severe that it almost felt as though I had not had the surgery at all and the only form of relief that I could achieve was from pain blocker injections in my lower back in the months that followed. Unfortunately, this wasn't a viable, long-term option as the injections are only effective for about seven days. In the end, I learnt to live with the pain, and it did lessen over time.

That was until I was about six months into writing this book, when some of my symptoms started to reemerge. I had been lucky to be honest. For the whole of 2020 I didn't have many bad days with my endo at all. There was the odd day here and there where I would experience some pain in my lower back but, on the whole, I was able to live a fairly normal, pain-free life. That all changed for me though at the start of 2021. Of course, even though I am writing a book to share my story in the hope of helping other women, I want to tell you that I made mistakes. I did what so many women do, I tried to ignore the symptoms and hoped they would go away on their own. I tried to ignore them as I didn't have the time to deal with it. I had things to do after all. I had a book to write!

Jokes aside, my point is that the journey to better physical and mental health and wellness is a neverending one. Mistakes are made along the way and that is totally okay. As they say, the first step is acknowledgement. The second step is to take action. Even small steps in the right direction count. And when you have bad days or weeks, recognize it, move on, and try to do better next time.

In the days when I was experiencing chronic pain, exhaustion, bloating and discomfort I became desperate for relief. The doctor that performed most of my other surgeries had said she felt my condition had reached a point where I needed more specialist care. I therefore decided I'd better try to see one of the specific endometriosis specialists in Los Angeles. The problem is that these doctors are rare, extremely difficult to get an appointment with, and consultations are incredibly expensive. And when I say expensive, I mean expensive. I called four so-called endo experts, three of whom had written books on the subject, and each were between $1,600 and $2,000 for a consultation! Not only is it almost impossible to get an appointment, but it is also completely unattainable for the average person due to the cost. I hate to think how much some of these specialists charge if a patient requires surgery. I was too scared to ask. I was told by one of the doctor's staff that if I paid a $2,000 deposit, I should be able to get in to see the doctor within about three months, so I pulled out my credit card and crossed my fingers, hoping for the best. I hung up after each call feeling deflated and thinking how awful it must be for the one in ten women globally, many of whom suffer in silence with no good options for help. This is the reality for most women suffering from the disease.

We desperately need more research into the disease so that better, less invasive testing methods can be developed, and better treatment options can be discovered. But research takes money. While more common than many other diseases, endometriosis has received relatively little research funding globally to support treatments and cures. In 2020, the U.S. Congress doubled the funding for endometriosis research to $26 million a year. It is definitely a move in the right direction, but more is needed, considering that it is a disease that affects so many women.

In Australia, the Australian Government Department of Health released a National Action Plan for Endometriosis, which included funding for research and development of better testing and treatment for the disease. This was largely implemented due to a push by Endometriosis Australia and Donna Ciccia, the founder of the organization. Endometriosis Australia also regularly campaigns through its Endo Warriors and other initiatives for funding for research. The organization also issues grants periodically for research.

FIBROIDS

Uterine fibroids are noncancerous growths of the uterus that often appear during childbearing years. Fibroids range in size, and in extreme cases can expand the uterus so that it reaches the rib cage and can add weight.

Some women have no symptoms but for those who do, the most common symptoms include:

- Heavy menstrual bleeding
- Menstrual periods lasting more than a week
- Pelvic pressure or pain
- Frequent urination
- Difficulty emptying the bladder
- Constipation
- Backache or leg pains.

Treatment options include medication and removal surgery. According to the Mayo Clinic[31], there are few known risk factors for uterine fibroids, other than being a woman of reproductive age. Factors that can have an impact on fibroid development include:

- **Race** – Although any woman of reproductive age can develop fibroids, black women are more likely to have fibroids than are women of other racial groups. In addition, black women have fibroids at younger ages, and they're also likely to have more or larger fibroids, along with more severe symptoms.
- **Heredity** – If your mother or sister had fibroids, you're at increased risk of developing them.
- **Other factors** – Onset of menstruation at an early age; obesity; vitamin D deficiency; having a diet higher in red meat and lower in green vegetables, fruit, and dairy; and drinking alcohol, including beer, appear to increase your risk of developing fibroids.

Fibroids can cause a person significant discomfort and fatigue from heavy blood loss. Fibroids can also cause infertility, pregnancy loss and pose risk of pregnancy complications.

---

31. https://www.mayoclinic.org/diseases-conditions/uterine-fibroids/symptoms-causes/syc-20354288

OVARIAN CYSTS

Ovarian cysts are fluid-filled sacs or pockets in an ovary or on its surface. Many women have ovarian cysts that do not present any symptoms and often resolve on their own without intervention. However, in some cases, ovarian cysts can cause pelvic pain (a sharp pain in the lower abdomen), uncomfortable fullness or heaviness in the abdomen and bloating. Ovarian cysts can also rupture, causing significant health issues.

A person's risk of developing an ovarian cyst increases due to the use of fertility drugs, as a result of pregnancy, for women who suffer from endometriosis and for those who experience a severe pelvic infection or if you have had a previous ovarian cyst, you are also at high risk of developing another. Additionally, cystic ovarian masses that develop after menopause can be cancerous.

UTERINE POLYPS

Uterine polyps are growths attached to the inner wall of the uterus that extend into the uterine cavity. Overgrowth of cells in the lining of the uterus (endometrium) leads to the formation of uterine polyps, also known as endometrial polyps. These polyps are usually noncancerous, although some can or can eventually turn into cancer (precancerous polyps).

Uterine polyps most commonly occur in women who are going through or are post-menopause. However, they can also occur in younger women and women who are prescribed tamoxifen, a drug therapy for breast cancer, are at high risk for development of uterine polyps.

Symptoms can include:
- Irregular menstrual bleeding
- Bleeding between menstrual periods
- Excessively heavy menstrual periods
- Vaginal bleeding after menopause
- Infertility.

POLYCYSTIC OVARIAN SYNDROME

Polycystic ovarian syndrome is a condition causing an imbalance of reproductive hormones that creates issues in the ovaries (including underdevelopment of eggs, irregular periods, and cysts in the ovaries) and metabolism problems. It is also one of the most common cause of infertility.

Polycystic ovarian syndrome is estimated to affect four to twenty percent of women of reproductive age worldwide.

FERTILITY ISSUES

Infertility can be defined as the inability to get pregnant after one year of trying to conceive. It affects an estimated fifteen percent of both men and women globally. For couples who have been trying to conceive for more than three years without success, the likelihood of getting pregnant naturally within the next year is approximately one in four.

In women, there can be many causes of infertility, including many of the conditions outlined in this chapter, including endometriosis, uterine fibroids, ovulation disorders, damage to fallopian tubes, cancers, and thyroid disease. The risk of infertility also increases as a person ages.

Infertility requires medical intervention, which can include medical treatments and medications, surgical procedures, and assisted conception such as intrauterine insemination (IUI) or in vitro fertilization (IVF). IUI is a form of artificial insemination whereby the sperm is washed and concentrated and then placed directly in a woman's uterus at the time when the ovary releases eggs to be fertilized. During IVF, eggs are removed during a surgical procedure generally following a period ranging from one to three weeks when a woman undertakes various tests and injects herself daily to help stimulate the ovaries to produce mature eggs. The success rates for both IUI and IVF range, depending on a woman's age, from four to fifty-four percent, but IVF is generally a lot more effective. The cost associated with IVF however, can be substantial. In the U.S., one cycle of IVF can be anywhere up to USD $20,000 or more. In Australia, costs can range between AUD $10,000 and $20,000 and in the U.K., costs range between £1,500 and £5,000 per cycle.

PREGNANCY LOSS

Pregnancy loss is a term that encompasses miscarriage, which is the loss of a pregnancy before twenty weeks, and late-term pregnancy loss. While the exact figures are unknown, it is estimated that between ten and twenty percent of pregnancies end in miscarriage. However, the figure is likely even higher, because many miscarriages occur so early in the pregnancy that the woman is unaware that they were pregnant.

Age can play a factor in miscarriage risk. As a woman ages, there is a higher chance of miscarriage in pregnancy, so as women are waiting longer to have children, this can be an additional hurdle. At age thirty-five, a woman has a twenty percent chance of miscarriage. By age forty, the risk increases to about forty percent and at age forty-five, it is about eighty percent.

Most miscarriages occur because the fetus is not developing properly, but not all. Sometimes miscarriages occur because a woman has another underlying health condition. This was my issue. I could get pregnant, but my body could not sustain a pregnancy. I continued to lose babies because in each pregnancy, I would develop cysts and those cysts would absorb all of the goodness that should have been feeding my baby. Instead, the cysts would grow, and my babies couldn't survive.

Even though miscarriage is common and many miscarriages occur within the first twelve weeks in a pregnancy, that doesn't lessen the pain and emotional and physical toll it can have on a woman. Most women who miscarry experience bleeding and pain or cramping in the abdomen or lower back. Additionally, most women get incredibly tired during the first trimester of a pregnancy and for a woman who experiences multiple miscarriages that are close together, this can be very difficult.

In most countries, there is no specific paid leave that a woman can access when she suffers a miscarriage, and this is something that needs to change. At Megaport Ltd, a company that I am on the board of, this is something we implemented for all our employees globally, because we recognize how difficult this is for people when they experience it and just how common it is. We want our employees to take time away from work to rest and recover physically and mentally without having to worry about work requirements or having to take unpaid leave (if they have no access to paid leave entitlements). I can tell you that the day that we rolled out the benefit, we were not flooded with requests for leave. It isn't something that has caused the organization a huge financial burden, but to the employees who have needed to access it, it has provided them with a great deal of comfort knowing that we care. I hope that more companies will consider following suit and not wait until the law dictates it.

PREGNANCY-RELATED HEALTH ISSUES

It is hard enough for some women to get pregnant, but the pregnancy itself can also be a risky business. There are many health issues that can occur during pregnancy for both the mother and the baby including:

- Iron deficiency anemia
- Gestational diabetes
- Depression and anxiety including post-natal depression
- Fetal problems
- High blood pressure
- Infections
- Hyperemesis gravidarum (severe morning sickness that can require hospitalization)
- Miscarriage
- Placenta previa
- Placental abruption
- Preeclampsia
- Preterm labor
- Breastfeeding issues such as inadequate milk supply, nipple and breast pain, mastitis (breast infection), yeast infection, bloody nipple discharge, blocked milk ducts, back pain, bruising, carpal tunnel, cramping.

FEMALE REPRODUCTIVE CANCERS

We have all heard about breast cancer statistics. Female breast cancer cases have now surpassed lung cancer cases globally with over two million new cases each year. Cancer is also the leading cause of death globally. There are also a number of gynecological cancers as well that start in a woman's reproductive organs or pelvis including:

- Cervical cancer
- Ovarian cancer
- Uterine cancer
- Vaginal cancer
- Vulvar cancer.

Each of these cancers present with different symptoms, requiring different treatments, including surgery, chemotherapy, and radiation. Each treatment option can further adversely impact a woman's health, as there are typically significant side-effects associated with some of the aggressive treatment options.

Any type of cancer in a man or a woman presents considerable challenges as they try to manage their day-to-day personal and professional responsibilities at the same time as dealing with this serious disease, which often requires extended periods of intensive treatment. However, just because a person has cancer and may be undergoing treatment, does not mean that they are incapable of performing their job or that they should be pushed aside or into another role. Employees with cancer all too often are subjected to discrimination because of perceptions around their ability to continue work and/or to perform while undergoing treatment. Like any illness, employees in many countries have certain protections, but there are ways to terminate their employment. In a restructure, for example, employers may find ways to move those employees along who simply no longer 'fit', because their personal situation poses a challenge.

Many employees who are diagnosed with cancer, particularly breast cancer, either want to or need to continue working through their treatment, and losing their employment can result in additional stress and detriment to their health. The John Hopkins Institute says that trying to understand and find ways to support these employees is not only important, but it is what is best for both the organization and the employee[32].

Employees that are able to continue working through treatment may require some flexibility for a period. Many managers though, don't understand the condition and don't know how to manage the employee or what to say. That's where the training of managers and access to information becomes important. The John Hopkins Institute has many great online resources available to assist both employers and managers to better support employees who have received a cancer diagnosis and importantly, as the Institute points out, this is an issue that impacts every employer. Just think about this: for every one hundred employees in the workplace, five will have a history of cancer, about 2.7percent will be in treatment for cancer and one in two men and one in three women will be diagnosed with a life-threatening form of cancer at some point in their lifetime.

MENOPAUSE

The last stage of a woman's reproductive life cycle is menopause. The average age of menopause is fifty-one. Menopause is defined as twelve months without a menstrual period and is often associated with hot flashes, headaches or migraines, night sweats, weight gain, loss of energy, brain fog or memory loss, anxiety attacks, dry skin and eyes, body aches and signs of estrogen deficiency including vaginal dryness, breast shrinkage, and urinary difficulty.

Significantly, the decline in estrogen associated with menopause can also increase the risk of heart attack, stroke, and osteoporosis, which accounts for the reason why one in three women as opposed to one in five men will suffer from osteoporosis in their lifetime. Symptoms can last on average anywhere from two years to ten years and for some women the effects, at times, can be debilitating. In some cases, so much so that it can amount to a disability that requires special accommodations or consideration of flexible work

---

32. https://www.johnshopkinssolutions.com/paying-attention-cancer-pays-off-employees/

arrangements by law. Until recently, menopause was not something that was discussed widely in the workplace context, because many women don't want to admit they are going through it for fear of repercussions – and men don't want to or don't know how to talk about it or deal with it. However, things are finally starting to change, and for good reason, and the issue of menopause is starting to get the attention and understanding that it deserves. In a report entitled Menopause transition: effects on women's economic participation[33], published in 2017, the Government Equalities Office in the U.K. recognized that increased rates of employment among women aged fifty and above mean that more working women than ever before will experience menopause transition during their working lives. It is also estimated that approximately twenty percent of the workforce globally (including approximately twenty-seven million employees in the U.S. each day) are suffering, often silently, with symptoms associated with menopause, and those that do disclose their symptoms are often labelled as emotional and unreliable. As Anne Loeher put it eloquently in her Fast Company article in 2016, How Menopause Silently Affects 27 Million Women At Work Every Day[34], "using a hot flash as a reason for forgetting something is tantamount to workplace suicide" and as Loeher points out, "even if you have a leader who's educated about menopause, she or he may end up fighting misinformation and lack the support it takes to find a solution".

Instead, many women simply leave the workforce. A 2019 survey conducted by global health insurance company BUPA and cited by the Chartered Institute of Personnel and Development, found that almost 900,000 women in the U.K. left their jobs over an undefined period of time because of menopausal symptoms[35]. With the high number of women who are experiencing menopause in practically every workplace, it is absolutely essential that employers find better ways to support women at this stage in their life. If we are ever to move closer towards closing the gender equality gap,

33. https://www.gov.uk/government/publications/menopause-transition-effects-on-womens-economic-participation

34. https://www.fastcompany.com/3056703/how-menopause-silently-affects-27-million-women-at-work-every-day

35. https://committees.parliament.uk/work/1416/menopause-and-the-workplace/

we simply cannot ignore this fundamental fact – that almost every woman will go through menopause, and most will experience the symptoms described above in the workplace as a result. It is becoming increasingly important for employers to be aware of the impacts of menopause on women at work, but awareness alone is simply not enough, because what we know is that most women are reluctant to talk about it. It is therefore equally important to provide a safe and supportive environment where women feel comfortable talking about menopause, as it is to train managers on how to manage employees with menopause-related symptoms and provide appropriate support and assistance. One effective way to do this is through employer-sponsored events or access to support groups.

The U.K. has started a 'menopause revolution' with some members of parliament putting menopause rights, entitlements, and education on the public agenda in 2019. Unfortunately, the move lost some of its momentum that was present early on, but I am pleased to hear that the U.K. government has called for input on the issue from legal groups, including the Employment Lawyers Association U.K.,[36] so that it can determine whether changes should be made to the law. I will watch keenly as the matter progresses and we start to see some of the debate emerge publicly. In Australia, a workplace menopause revolution is also happening, but on a smaller scale. Many business networks and female support groups are starting to talk more about the issue. I hosted a women's health event with the Victorian Government in 2019, which was attended by hundreds of women and one of the topics that we focused on was menopause in the workplace. I had so many women lining up after the event to speak with me and have been contacted by many women since, all wanting more discussion, and more to be done about this issue. People are starting to demand that employers pay more attention, and that they start taking action.

One such organization in Australia that has assisted in leading this charge is the Australian based employee benefits platform, Circle

---

36. https://www.elaweb.org.uk/

In[37]. In 2021, they released a report which was supported by the Victorian Women's Trust[38] called Driving the change: Menopause and the workplace[39]. Through their research, which included the input of approximately 700 women, they have determined that globally "there is a culture of ignorance and isolation around menopause in the workplace, and a glaring lack of support for employees and their managers."[40] They are but one organization who wants to see change, and their research found that more than half of the respondents that had experienced menopause said managing work during their menopausal transition was "challenging" and eighty-three percent said their work was negatively affected. Interestingly, seventy-six percent said they would have benefitted from information, advice, and support at work. In contrast, the U.S. is unfortunately rather behind on the issue of menopause at work, with few examples of companies that are taking active steps to specifically support employees who are experiencing the symptoms associated with menopause in the workplace.

There are many ways employers can break down the taboo surrounding menopause and start better supporting their female population. Education is a key piece of the puzzle. Managers should be educated on the impacts of menopause on a woman, specifically how this might affect her experiences at work, and ways that the manager and the organization can support her. Flexibility in hours and working arrangements, and offering leave entitlements that are catered more appropriately to women who are experiencing severe menopause symptoms are also equally valuable.

As many organizations are beginning to recognize the impact of fertility issues and miscarriage on employees and their careers, employers should also be equally considering similar issues surrounding menopause and how to best to support more mature, experienced workers to succeed during this time of their lives as

---

37. https://circlein.com/

38. https://www.vwt.org.au/

39. https://circlein.com/resources/driving-the-change-menopause-and-the-workplace/

40. *Driving the change: Menopause and the workplace*, Circle In, page 2.

well. Similarly, many employers have employee wellness programs and initiatives focused on stress, mental health and physical fitness including sessions on weight loss, yoga and dealing with addictions such as smoking, etc. Employers should also consider holding similar sessions or programs that are focused on some less typical topics, such as fertility challenges, pregnancy loss and menopause.

Providing counselling, support groups such as Menopause Chicks[41] to share experiences and ideas and providing tools such as desk fans, a change room (so that employees can change in peace without having to squeeze into a toilet cubical) or even access to cold water, ice or ice-blocks are all things that can really assist. As a first step though, having a policy that confirms the company's commitment to supportive and open conversations on menopause and its impacts at work, which also outlines the type of support that is available and how and to who employees can raise issues, is an incredibly important first step.

THE EFFECTS AT WORK

In addition to the physical impacts of the many female health issues, we simply cannot ignore the significant psychological impacts of infertility, child loss and the other diseases and health conditions that impact women. The impacts to mental health can be the most difficult side-effect for many women and can cause anxiety, depression, feelings of hopelessness or worthlessness, low self-esteem, diminished motivation, guilt, severe distress, and reduced quality of life. For some women, it means the loss of opportunity, the loss of life plans and dreams. Social, cultural, and individual factors also play a part in the type of support and resources that a woman experiencing a health issue or child loss will have access to and this too can significantly impact her quality of life. When a woman experiences these types of difficulties, the stress and other psychological impacts can cause other health conditions, or

---

41. http://www.menopausechicks.com/

exacerbate existing ones. This has definitely been true for me. When I was in London, I was under so much stress working nights that it caused me to experience an increase in the severity of my endometriosis symptoms and the more stressed I was, the more unwell I would become. It also impacted my general health; I ended up with a flu that turned into pneumonia, which I could not shake for about three months. It can become a vicious cycle. You need to rest to get well and the more you rest, the more stressed you can become about the work that is not being completed and the commitments that you are not keeping.

Not only can it have a severe impact on quality of life, but all of the health issues that women experience every single day can end up impacting both personal and professional relationships as well as a woman's career prospects. As so many women have told me time and again, they were forced out of jobs, they left because they felt that they had no option, or they were unable to manage the demands of the job or the workplace and obtain the treatment needed to manage their condition because they simply weren't supported or provided with flexibility to be able to do both.

I can almost hear some people now saying, "Yeah, but I am an employer, and I am hiring this person to do a job. I can't just be flexible all the time. It simply isn't possible". Believe me, I get it. I absolutely acknowledge and agree that sometimes it just isn't possible to say, you can work from home or work nights, for example. If an employee is a customer representative working in your physical store, that person cannot serve customers from their sofa! It is true that maybe in those types of situations, that is not the right role for that person.

However, what I also know is that those situations are not the norm. There are far more situations where employers can find ways to offer assistance, support and flexibility to employees and there are ways to try to work with your employees to find a middle ground solution. Not every answer needs to be yes. It just needs to be, "We can't do that but let's try to find another solution to assist you". And sometimes it might also be, "Let's work towards that goal and here are the steps that we can take to get there together". As someone who has had her fair share of challenges, managing some severe symptoms associated with health conditions, just hearing a manager say these words and knowing they genuinely want to try to work with you to find a way to assist you to continue to succeed means all the difference. It can directly impact a person's mental health which, I am absolutely certain, has a positive impact on a person's recovery and is connected to the severity of the symptoms a person may experience as a result of their health condition. If you have ever had a day when you have received terrible news or something bad has happened but you meet up with a friend or sit with a loved one and pour your heart out, possibly over a glass of wine or two, and that person is supportive and loving and tells you it's going to be okay and that they are there for you, then you will know exactly what I mean. Having someone to listen and support you usually makes big problems seem smaller and a lot more manageable, not to mention that two minds working through a challenge often produces a better result as well.

Uncomfortable Conversations

Why don't more women speak up in the workplace when they are experiencing fertility challenges, pregnancy loss and health issues that are impacting them at work? There are many reasons, but fear and stigma rank high on the list. Women are often fearful that they will appear weak, that they are not up to the demands or pressures of the job or that they are simply incapable or unreliable.

I can't count the number of women who have told me stories over the years about being looked over for a promotion, being removed from an account or denied an opportunity after experiencing issues related to immediate family, pregnancy, childcare responsibilities or their health. Women are therefore often fearful of the consequences of raising these issues with their employers and the reality, unfortunately, is that their fear is often justified. There remains a stigma attached to these issues in so far as they relate to the workplace. I have spoken to board members, CEOs, executive teams, and human resources professionals about managing employee matters around these types of issues. Over the years, I have spoken to thousands of people through the work that I do and I can tell you that more often than not, the employee who raises a health issue or says that they cannot fulfill a requirement due to their parental responsibilities is the one that is eliminated from a selection process for a new role, promotion or opportunity because it is that same employee that is not quite as 'committed' as the others in the selection pool.

There is, unfortunately, quite obviously a negative perception of those who have a life outside of the workplace if the responsibilities associated with that life are seen to impact the employee at work. That kind of age-old belief and the negative connotations that follow are extremely difficult to break and we all have them to some extent, in one area or another. We all have implicit bias, and we all hold views and ideas about certain things, some of which we may not even be conscious of. For me, one of the things I realized about myself was that I was unconsciously judgmental of other women who didn't push through and keep going. If an employee said they were sick and needed time off work for the flu or an ear infection for example, I would silently think, "For goodness sake! It's just the flu. I have had surgery in a morning and been back at my laptop by the afternoon". My own bias was such that I would think negatively about another person if they needed time off work to heal, because I never took any time to do that for myself. I was very wrong. I was unfairly judgmental, and I was probably also very jealous, because I really did want to take time to rest.

How many times have you personally experienced or heard words about someone else such as, "Are you sure this is the right place for you?", "It's just not the right time for that promotion", "She's not the right cultural fit for the organization", or "I am not sure she is really committed", when a person asks for workplace flexibility such as a move to part-time hours, a change in working hours or asks for an extended leave due to illness or injury, pregnancy, parental or carer responsibilities?

Unfortunately, this is all too common. Many of the employers I have worked with over the years haven't even recognized that the reason they hold this view might actually be related back to the employee's health issue, family responsibilities or request for flexibility or leave. However, in so many cases, it has been clear to me, based on the information I have been presented with, that these things have directly played a part in the events that have transpired and the formulation of the company's views about the individual.

The first step towards change for all of us is recognizing the areas where we might have these types of biases or views, and starting to work on implementing change in how we perceive others. The only way to do that is to first recognize that we are wrong, and most importantly why we are wrong, and then work out ways to actively change our thinking. Working out the 'why' is an incredibly important part of this process, because without understanding why we have the views and why they are wrong, outdated or perhaps not applicable to everyone or every situation, it is difficult for us to find a purpose and commit to change.

In my situation, once I recognized that I had a bias, I realized I needed to change my own life and my responses to managing my own health conditions because not doing so was continuing to impact my health, my personal relationships, and my work. It made me exhausted and resentful, and I was not performing at my best as a result. That became my 'why' because it formed the basis of the incorrect views I had about others and why I needed to take active steps to change them. The way that I did that was by speaking out, listening to others' experiences and needs and then actively implementing ways to better support people in the organizations that I am fortunate to be a part of.

I am not going to lie to you though – that initial conversation when you first raise these issues for consideration on a board, with an executive team or with a group of managers or human resources professionals can be tough, especially if it is far removed from anything that has ever been considered a part of your workplace. The first time I raised these issues at a board meeting there was some awkward silence, followed by some debate about whether or not this was a conversation that had a place within the workplace and whether opening the proverbial can of worms was something that we wanted to do. For me, it was obviously a 'hell yes!' but keeping in mind the biases and views that everybody has about these issues, that is unlikely to be the response you will get from every single person in a meeting.

Implementing change and challenging ideas and views is something that takes time and doesn't typically happen overnight. However, just because something is difficult or because you are likely to be faced with opposing views, that certainly doesn't mean that we shouldn't try. Starting the conversation is the first step. My advice though, is to be armed with a plan, and that requires ensuring you do some preparation and research. For me, this included the following steps:

- Identify the **issues;**
- Determine the **impact** of the issues on the organization;
- Look at what **other companies** in the industry are doing;
- Find some **examples** of companies that have implemented policies and benefits in this space effectively and who have had success;

- Develop some **options**;
- Determine **costings**;
- Formulate a **timeline**;
- Make **recommendations** for implementation. Tip: it is often better to stagger the implementation over time. If these are new ideas, don't ask for the entire wish list all at once. Results generate trust, belief in the strategy/plan and generally greater **flexibility** – so be prepared to start small if needed and increase over time as you show that the plan is working!

The good news is that more often than not, that first conversation is the most difficult to have because you can be faced with awkward silence, strong opposing views and even looks of disbelief that these topics are being discussed in the workplace. Of the three, I am not sure which is worse, but I do know with some certainty that almost every time, the conversation changes, develops and improves over time. People are often uncomfortable and express some shock and pushback against change. However, once you start introducing ideas and challenging perceptions, most importantly, through linking it back to the research, science, and statistics that back up your proposals, people start to listen more and think about your ideas.

Being armed with the data to back up your proposal is absolutely critical though, because if you open an initial discussion without having done your research first, you will have a hard time getting the same people to listen to you a second time once they realize the topic that you want to talk about. However, if you are prepared to make your arguments and link them back to the business case in that first meeting, people are more likely to listen to you the next time you raise the issues for consideration.

You don't have to be perfect, but it is important to appear credible and understand that not everyone has the same agenda and the same objectives. I may want to create a workplace where everyone's differences are valued, respected and supported in every single way possible; but to a certain extent those goals may conflict with the goals of shareholders in a public company who want to see a profitable return on their investment. Now I understand (and hopefully you do as well, after reading this book!) that looking after employees generates more loyal, productive employees, but at the same time, I also understand that the company is in the business of making a profit for its shareholders. It is not a philanthropic organization in the business of looking after employees, as nice as that would be. So, as such, a balance must be found that appropriately addresses the needs of both the shareholders and the employees, so that they are ultimately able to perform at their best..

When I walk into meetings to discuss a change to employee benefits, the introduction of a policy, or a new initiative to better support our employees at work, I am always armed with the information, the statistics, the research, a competitor overview, some options, and costs and, finally, my recommendations. If possible, I also try to prepare an analysis that demonstrates the cost versus benefit ratios, because an argument becomes considerably more compelling where you are able to show "if we spend $X per employee on this, then we are likely to see an $Y increase in Z". The other thing I do is try to anticipate the opposition so that I am not caught off guard and I am prepared to counterargue. This also assists with credibility and this type of preparation paves the way for future discussions if you aren't able to get the approvals you are seeking the first time around.

Don't get disheartened if you don't get the response you are seeking the first time. If you are prepared with good arguments and you have done your research, you establish credibility regardless. No one thinks poorly of someone who has prepared well and has good ideas. That doesn't always mean you will gain agreement with your propositions or approval of your proposals, but you are likely to generate the respect of those who are listening and sometimes it is the first step in the process towards implementing a change. I have presented proposals in many meetings where they have been considered and debated but sometimes, I am told "Not yet", "We are not quite ready" or "We want to watch this/consider this/gather more data", and that's okay. I never see this as a "no". I see that as progress towards change. So, when we look at the reasons why it is important to support women in the workplace who are experiencing challenges such as fertility issues, associated health problems and pregnancy loss, it is important to understand why having an inclusive and supportive environment is important. We know with some certainty that statistically, women bear more of the household and childcare responsibilities globally; women generally have more responsibility for the care of loved ones including elderly parents; women are more likely to end up single mothers with the primary care of children and women suffer more health issues than men. Also, women are more likely to retire single without spouse support, and that can impact a woman's career decisions.

We also know the extremely high percentages of women that suffer miscarriage every day. The loss of a pregnancy during the first thirteen weeks of pregnancy (the first trimester) is called early pregnancy loss or miscarriage and it is estimated to occur in between ten to twenty percent of pregnancies globally. This means that on any day, there is a high chance that someone in your workplace may be impacted by fertility struggles or miscarriage. However, most employers are ill-equipped to support an employee who is returning to work following a pregnancy loss. Managers are rarely trained appropriately on managing employee illness, injury or health issues generally – let alone something as specific and sensitive as pregnancy loss and fertility issues. There are also few organizations that have appropriate policies and procedures to support an employee that is dealing with these issues.

People often don't know what to say to a person who has suffered a pregnancy loss or how to even approach a person who is returning from leave following this type of experience. Unfortunately, what typically happens is that the employee is either ignored for fear of saying the wrong thing, or people actually do end up saying awkward or insensitive things. We are all human and these types of situations can be incredibly challenging to manage, both as an employee communicating with a colleague and as a manager that has a staff member who has experienced such a loss. For every person, the support they need or want will be different as well, but there are things that every employer and every manager can do to prepare for each situation as it arises.

One thing should be absolutely clear – when an employee suffers a pregnancy loss, there is grieving, and healing required. Employees can feel lost and alone and even if they do not want to talk about it or do not want to ask for, or even access any support, making it available and letting the person know you care and that the support is there if needed, is a crucial part of the road to recovery.

The Pink Elephants Network is an organization that provides support and resources for those who are suffering from fertility issues or who have experienced miscarriage. The organization created the Leave for Loss campaign, which ultimately resulted in the Australian Federal Government introducing legislation to provide employees in Australia with paid leave following a miscarriage. As part of the campaign, the organization has undertaken research around the impact of fertility issues in the workplace and, as stated on their website, "Miscarriage and infertility can induce an intense period of emotional distress and if left unsupported, can lead to heightened anxiety symptoms and/or depression." The aim of the organization is to assist employers to support their employees who are experiencing fertility and child loss.

Many employees feel unable to speak up when they are experiencing fertility issues or pregnancy loss, especially when it occurs within the first trimester, as most people do not disclose publicly that they are pregnant until they pass the first three months of pregnancy. It can therefore be incredibly difficult for an employee to speak out to their employer and explain that they need support and time to grieve and heal. One of the problems is that many people hold a belief, whether conscious or not, that the early loss of a pregnancy is not as bad as a full-term stillbirth.

When I lost my baby, one of my closest friends who had a sister that had lost her baby at birth said something to me that to this day pierces my heart every time that I think about it. She said, "Your experience is nothing like my sister. How dare you compare your situation to hers when she had a baby that she gave birth to and held before he passed away." There is no hierarchy of loss. Grief is overwhelming and sad for everyone who experiences it. As Oprah Winfrey said in the 2021 documentary *The Me You Can't*

See,[42] "Grief is the loss of anything that matters". Unfortunately, though, the view expressed by my friend that day is not uncommon, and her reaction was unsurprising, as so many people do hold these types of beliefs when it comes to pregnancy loss.

What I know from my own experience is that fertility treatments, miscarriage and the surgery that can sometimes follow a pregnancy loss are all things that take a toll on a person's body and mind and time is needed to heal both. Even those women who can take the emotional aspect of the experience and place it inside a box to be dealt with later, still need time for their body to heal physically. I didn't take that time, and ultimately my health suffered. It is completely unrealistic to think that any woman could experience a pregnancy loss, have a dilation and curettage (a procedure to remove the uterine lining after a miscarriage) under general anesthesia and then return to work immediately and perform at their full potential. Yet, across the globe, we have required women to do this for a long time.

In March 2021, New Zealand became one of the first countries to legalize leave for women who experience miscarriage. In Australia, thanks to the Pink Elephants Network and those who have campaigned for the Leave for Loss cause, legislation was introduced into Australian parliament in June to amend the Fair Work Act 2009 (Cth) and provide paid leave for any employee experiencing miscarriage. Other countries with legislation of this kind include the Philippines and India, where women are entitled to six weeks of paid leave if they miscarry. But the law applies only to those who work at a company with ten people or more. In Britain, women are entitled to paid leave if they have a miscarriage or stillborn birth after twenty-four weeks. The United States has no laws addressing miscarriages or stillborn births in regards to the workplace.

Women in some countries might have the ability to simply call in sick and utilize whatever ordinary sick leave benefits they have, but for others this has not been possible and, as many of the

---

42. https://tv.apple.com/us/show/the-me-you-cant-see/umc.cmc.4amwght1qtt8ioilwr0mgnf6d?ctx_brand=tvs.sbd.4000&ign-itsc-g=MC_20000&ign-itsct=atvp_brand_omd&mttn3pid=Google%20AdWords&mttnagencyid=a5e&mttncc=US&mttn-siteid=143238&mttnsubad=OUS2019901_1-525911408545-c&mttnsubkw=123936717315_f54oi2Iv_&mttnsubplmnt=

campaigners for early pregnancy loss leave in New Zealand and Australia have pointed out, grieving for the loss of a child is not an illness. It is a major life event that is certainly not akin to a cold or flu. It is something quite different, so why should an employee be forced to access their sick leave in the circumstances? We desperately need more countries around the world to follow the examples of the countries that have taken the initiative to introduce these types of benefits and we also need employers globally to be proactive, not to simply sit back and wait for the law to regulate in this area and introduce policies that support employees that experience pregnancy loss to take time away from work to rest and heal.

Those who are fortunate enough to be in situations where they are not living paycheck to paycheck, have an obligation to stand up and speak up on behalf of all of those women who are unable to do so, because they live in fear of stepping out of line and risking their livelihood. I want to dispel a myth right now. Those of us who speak up are not fearless. If you wait for a time when there is no fear, you will never speak up. You will never act. Starting conversations to create change can be difficult, and most people walk into meetings with some fear when addressing such new or novel ideas. Fear challenges us though, and gives us adrenalin to push through boundaries and strive for improvements.

Leaders have a job to do: to disrupt the status quo where change is needed. That takes courage, but it is often still done with some fear and that's okay. That is just a part of being human. We all have the right to speak up and ask for change in every aspect of life if change is needed. Silence serves no one. The workplace is an institution that has been built on age-old ideas and as we grow and develop as a species and strive towards more equality within the workplace, diversity and inclusion, know that you have the right to speak up and start demanding more, not just as employees but as customers as well. Speaking up and demanding change comes in many different forms as I have outlined in **So, What Can You Do?**

We can ask our employers for better support, better benefits and policies and we can speak as consumers as well when we make choices about which companies to support. Just like employees, customers are increasingly demanding more of their service providers. In the legal industry, we are seeing this more and more as clients increasingly want to know what our male versus female partner and lawyer ratios are, how diverse our lawyers are and what our strategies are for striving to continually improve.

Speaking up also comes in the form of action, by setting appropriate boundaries. Most women need to get better at setting boundaries. I did an incredibly poor job of this until relatively recently and even now I still struggle with this from time to time. I am always actively working on it and striving to improve. It is important to consider that the human brain often conceives the worst-case scenario whenever we are faced with a difficult situation. Many of us spend hours going back and forth in our minds over all of the possibilities and often revert to the worst-case option – but equally the reverse is possible, and you will never know what the outcome will be until you have the conversation, ask for the help or raise the issue in your workplace. It is important to think about this and to try to adopt this positive mindset, armed with the data and options of course, when entering these types of discussions.

Looking at it from an employer's point of view, there are a few things that they will want to understand, one of which is the legal risk. This is an important aspect of any discussion around employee health, fertility issues, pregnancy loss and child or family responsibilities, because there are strict privacy and discrimination laws that apply in most countries. We are not all lawyers, and most people will not be able to advise on this, but it is nonetheless an important consideration to factor into any discussion, especially when seeking to introduce new policies, benefits, support programs or wellness initiatives in the workplace. Obtaining legal advice and assistance throughout the implementation is therefore a cost that may need to be factored into your proposal when presenting your ideas for discussion.

It is going to be crucial to prepare and present the business case well, but at the end of the day, there is obviously a human element to the discussion which should not be undervalued. Importantly, while providing better support for your employees is a good thing to do for your people, ultimately it has positive benefits for the organization as well, in all of the ways that I discuss throughout this book. Looking at the benefits to the individual though, let's focus on conversations and sharing for a moment.

I couldn't share my story the day after each event in my life happened. It took time for me to reach a point in my life where I felt like my story should be shared so openly, warts and all, in the hope that it might assist others. However, despite that, there were certainly people that I did disclose bits and pieces to as I felt comfortable doing so and there were people in my life, including within my workplace, who made me feel supported as I did so. There were people who would just listen, others who would offer me different types of support or advice, and those who shared their own stories with me as well. This helped immensely to get me through particularly difficult times and, like many other women, sharing my story with other women who understood what I was going through was a form of healing itself. When I suffered pregnancy loss after pregnancy loss and I was desperately wanting to be part of the 'mommy' community, it gave me another community to be a part of – a sense of belonging to an invisible group of women who also wore the scars of deep wounds inflicted as a result of the loss of a pregnancy, a child, motherhood and a dream.

Talking about experiences and giving people the space to share establishes mutual trust through shared experiences and this in turn helps to normalize the topic and assist people to forge a path onwards through community connection. This is equally true for men and women. Women carry the burden of their body not working in the way that they had hoped it would, the loss of a child, the loss of hope and often a lack of understanding why – while men bear witness to their loved one who is suffering physically and mentally, while they too carry their own feelings of loss and sometimes failure as well.

Finding a community of people who understand can be an essential part of a person's healing process. When Meghan Markle, the Duchess of Sussex wrote openly about her pregnancy loss in the *New York Times* piece, 'The Losses We Share'[43], women from all over

---

43. https://www.nytimes.com/2020/11/25/opinion/meghan-markle-miscarriage.html

the world praised her for speaking out about such a personal issue as it gave other women a sense of belonging and understanding. Her message in that article was clear: "Perhaps the path to healing begins with three simple words: Are you OK?", but more than that, being prepared to really listen to the answer with an open heart and mind. I would also go a step further. Employers should also be presenting options to support their employees, because people will commonly ask a person if they are okay and receive an automatic "I'm fine", response. Presenting an offer to assist, *and* options is far more likely to result in an employee seeking the assistance and support that they need.

As the Duchess points out, "Losing a child means carrying an almost unbearable grief, experienced by many, but talked about by few". In speaking out about her own experience, the Duchess touched other women and gave them the confidence to share their own experiences and let others know that they may not be okay. Similarly, other public personalities such as Michelle Obama, Beyoncé, Christina Perry and Chrissy Teigen have also talked publicly about their experiences of losing a baby and their stories have generated similar reactions, with people thanking them for speaking out about the issue in the hope of debunking the taboo surrounding the topic.

Providing employees with a safe and supportive environment to speak up and let an employer know when they are experiencing health issues, fertility problems or pregnancy loss, in my view, is essential. However, these types of conversations involve highly sensitive and personal information and therefore they must be conducted appropriately and voluntarily. One of the worst things a person can experience at work is the dreaded questioning about children from coworkers when the questions are unwanted and have the potential to cause pain. Discussions about family, children and fertility in the workplace can be difficult for many employees.

Think about employee lunches, work social events and Friday night drinks where talk between colleagues typically turns to family life at some point during conversations. People naturally ask one another whether they have a partner, whether they are married and if they have any children, and often solicit answers to seemingly innocent questions that can cause feelings of intense grief in a person who is experiencing the pain associated with the loss of a child or problems conceiving.

One of the things that I myself often found was that when I didn't yet have children and my response was, "No", the next question would be something like, "Don't you want kids?" or "Do you think that you'll have them some day?" as if it's that easy a choice as simply wanting children or not. This is something that people do outside of the workplace as well, of course. However, in the outside world we can excuse ourselves from a situation, go home or decide not to engage in a conversation with that person. In the workplace context that is often not possible, and if a person does refuse to respond, ask others to change the subject or excuse themselves from a conversation, they may be viewed as rude, angry, unprofessional, or not a team-player. As Samantha Jones from the 1990s hit television show *Sex and the City* said, "A guy gets angry in a meeting he's a pistol. A woman, she's emotional". It's a stereotype that unfortunately is still often applied even today.

In workplace social settings, questions are often asked of people who do not partake in the consumption of alcoholic drinks. For an employee that is trying to conceive, undergoing fertility treatments or an employee who is pregnant, these questions can be difficult and upsetting, as they can be a trigger to a person who is stressed and anxious about what might be an already difficult process. Alcohol has become a large part of the social culture in many countries and studies have shown that those who do not drink are stigmatized at times by being made to feel as those they have departed from the 'acceptable social norm'.

An employee who is not drinking while trying to conceive or pregnant also faces this same issue if they are not comfortable disclosing the reason they are electing not to consume alcohol. Even employees who already have children can face similar stresses in the workplace if they are experiencing difficulties conceiving another child, because so often during these same social conversations over the water cooler an employee will ask questions such as, "Do you want any more children?", "How many children do you think you will have?" or "Do you want to try for a boy/girl?"

So, what is the solution? Well, education of employees and managers is a key component and something that is often lacking within organizations. In my years of work in the area of employment law, I have seen many companies that just train their employees to the minimum extent required by law and others that do little or no training at all, sometimes just briefly during induction and only covering a basic, "Here are our policies. They prohibit discrimination.... etc." I think that employers miss opportunities by failing to invest resources in the training of their workforce on a regular basis. But one training is certainly not equal to the next. For any training to be effective and worthwhile, it needs to be done well. It should be informative, educational, engaging and ultimately test the knowledge of the attendees, as this is the best way to learn content.

Training can serve a few very useful purposes. Firstly, when done well, it demonstrates to employees that this is an organization that really cares and is invested in its people. It is not an organization that merely wants to tick a metaphorical compliance box. Secondly, it can educate employees and provide managers with strategies, tools, and resources to more effectively support their employees through a range of issues, and it also assists to reduce an organization's legal risk. When managers are armed with the tools they need to handle employee issues as and when they arise and they are provided with the ability to upskill in these areas, it inevitably reduces the risk of employee claims for mishandling of matters related to employee health issues, leave periods, parental responsibilities, pregnancy loss and many other matters.

Encouraging your employees to be open about any health, fertility, or family challenges they might be suffering also helps an organization to better plan ahead and avoid any pitfalls. For example, if an organization provides employees with the support that they need to come forward when they experience a pregnancy loss, the company can allocate work accordingly and ultimately the employee is not at risk of a negative perception that they have failed to perform at the required standard by not being able to submit a piece of work or meet a project deadline. Being silent is rarely a good option when a person is experiencing something that is impacting their work, because ultimately an employer is entitled to assess a person's work based on the facts at hand, and if an employer remains in the dark as to any personal issues that someone may be experiencing, it can lead to performance concerns or even formal performance management or termination in some cases.

Conversations about health, fertility and mental health issues can be difficult for anyone. Talking about these issues and being open to receiving this type of information from your employees so that you can better understand how to support them in the workplace is a crucial component of the workplace gender gap discussion. If we don't start to have these types of conversations in workplaces, we are missing a fundamental piece of the puzzle, because the fact is that **women experience these types of issues in their lives every single day** and the effects simply don't stop once the person enters the workplace or logs onto their computer.

Some people might be able to push through for a period, like I did, but ultimately that just isn't sustainable. It is a bit like walking across a tightrope. You will wobble and bob up and down for a while, desperately trying to keep at least a toe on that rope at all times. Eventually though, you slip, come crashing down and you just might break a few valuable things in the process. I know I did.

Your Stories

Over the years when I have shared my story with women and have explained why I believe that change needs to happen within almost every workplace, many of those women have told me their stories as well. It seems to me that no matter where I turn, there are women with their own experiences of unfair treatment or unsupportive workplaces or managers. I can think of so many of my own friends and family who have suffered in the workplace with health conditions or child loss, and I can recall many examples of awful treatment that people I know have been subjected to. If I was to write about each and every one of those experiences, I don't think I would ever have finished this book, because there are examples of women being ill treated in workplaces around the world every single day.

However, instead, I put a call out and asked for women who wanted to share their stories to come forward. Some of these women are strangers and many have never shared their stories, at least not publicly. I think it is important to hear from these women because I am quite sure that almost everyone reading this will be able to relate to at least some parts of their stories and it shows you and them that none of us are alone in this, but change is important for all of us. So, I thank each one of them for letting us into such personal and painful memories.

SARAH - UNITED STATES

It was 2012, and I was a thirty-three year-old employment lawyer and senior associate, working my way up the corporate ladder and dreaming of the baby my partner and I were looking forward to adding to our family.

In the first few months, everything had been going well. However, at my twenty-week scan, I was delivered the devastating news that there was something wrong with my baby's heart. Although the nurse wasn't qualified to diagnose exactly what was happening, I knew from her panicked voice and the fumbling of her words that it was serious.

On that afternoon, as I exited out of the testing facility with a referral for a specialist, I was faced with a wall of uncertainty and anxiety. Not only did I have my baby's health to worry about, but I'd just been hit with a bill for $5000 – just for the scan and heart testing. And now, I had to go back to work and paste a smile on; pretend that all was okay. In my industry, empathy was rarely given or displayed, but as a female employee, I felt it was even more imperative that I keep this news to myself. The last thing I wanted was to be seen as the 'overly emotional' and 'fragile' woman in the office.

After all, 'emotional' was the exact word that management had labelled me over the past few months. The reason? Because one of my close colleagues had died. I remember shortly after her death, I'd been called in for a performance review and they'd made a big deal about how stressed I'd been, before adding as an afterthought, "Oh, I guess that could just be because of Maxine's death?"

There was just no room for an 'overly emotional woman' in our firm, and I didn't want to do anything to add to these stereotypes.

On top of all of this, I was already facing discrimination in the workplace simply for being pregnant. There was a perception that I was no longer 'capable' because I was expecting a child – especially when I opted for caution with things like lifting heavy boxes. All of these things made me feel less inclined to open up to my workplace about how much I was struggling emotionally.

Despite all of this, I continued to excel at work, taking on more and more caseloads – all the while trying desperately to get an appointment with my obgyn or another specialist to find out what could be done for our baby.

Eventually, I was able to get an appointment with a medical expert at UCFS Medical Center, which specialized in children's hearts, as well as a Stanford specialist. Unfortunately, the more appointments I needed, the longer I was delayed from knowing whether there was a chance at saving my baby's life, or if I'd need to have a termination. Knowing that I may have to abort this precious child who was growing bigger and bigger with every day that passed – as I struggled desperately to find answers – only created more trauma and anxiety within me. Worst of all, there were few people I could speak to about what was happening.

Abortion itself is a highly emotional and loaded topic, and one that elicits very strong opinions and feelings – but when it comes to late terminations, the judgement is even stronger. People assume that any woman who ends her pregnancy after twenty weeks is getting rid of the baby for no other reason than convenience. At best, it's seen as unethical, at worst, you're a murderer. Yet, none of these labels fitted me or the situation I was in. I wanted this child. I didn't want to terminate; and if I was advised to, I wanted to ensure it was done as soon as possible. Yet, the delay in medical treatment and advice, meant that – if I were to require a termination, or it was advised – I would automatically fall within the 'late-term abortion' category.

Eventually, at twenty-three weeks of pregnancy, a specialist appointment was scheduled and I was delivered the news. My baby only had half a heart. Not only that, but the ventricles weren't working as they should, and there was no way to repair them. With sadness in her own eyes, the female specialist sat me down and drew a picture of my baby's heart, before looking me in the eyes and sadly stating: "Sarah, I fight for many of these babies every day, but due to the severe nature of your baby's heart issues, yours is one that I cannot fight for."

It was at this moment that I realized that, as a mother, this was the first big choice I had to make for my child. It was devastating, and yet, also one that had to be made out of love. My partner and I knew that if our baby made it to birth, he would be in immense pain, and that keeping him alive would be a decision that benefited only us. We were totally heartbroken. Even at this early stage I had already been feeling kicks, and we so wanted to welcome this child into the world.

Due to the fact that I was now four months into pregnancy, a termination was now no longer possible in my city. So, on top of the grief that I was already experiencing, I had to arrange to fly to L.A. to see a doctor who was willing to perform a late-term procedure. However, this took time – meaning that, my baby continued to grow and kick inside of me. Every day, as I felt those little flutters and bumps, I was filled with devastation.

After the procedure, I told people at work I'd lost the baby. It was too hard to describe everything that had happened, and what I was going through. As a result, people assumed it was a miscarriage, and when this happened, I didn't immediately correct them. I was worried about the stigma and even potential violence from people I didn't know. I'd heard from my doctor that she'd had threats and seen protesters who had literally attacked women or staff as they entered or exited abortion clinics. All of this left me feeling very alone in my journey, and unable to open up to any of my management team about what I was going through, nor to ask about what options were available to me in terms of leave.

In the end, I took a week off. In hindsight, it just wasn't enough time. The body needs time to heal after something so traumatic, but I didn't want to be seen as incompetent. I wanted to be a team player, and taking additional time off would have only made me look bad.

For the most part, my managers responded very awkwardly. No one knew what to say or how to talk about the issue. Coming back to work was difficult in many different ways. Not only was I bleeding heavily after the procedure, but my milk also came in. It was traumatic to walk around the office every day looking so noticeably pregnant, yet having no baby.

One of my female partners tried to be understanding, but no real options of support were offered to me. In my state of grief and distress, it would have been enormously helpful to have someone say, "Sarah, you should take some time off", or, "Let me help you look into what leave you're entitled to". I really needed someone to tell me what was available, and to assist me with managing my workload before/afterwards – instead of leaving me to figure it out.

Whilst my firm did have benefits and policies in place that could have helped me through this time (including a short-term disability policy), I was not aware of everything I had access to. As someone who had just ended their pregnancy and was grieving, I needed someone to tell me what they were and what was available. I just didn't have the mental bandwidth to advocate for myself.

Instead, I constantly felt that I needed to prove myself, and that if I didn't, my career would be in jeopardy. At no time did anyone reassure me that I was a valued employee, or that my progression within our workplace wouldn't be impacted by taking time off.

Shortly after returning from my seven days of leave, I was thrust into working fifty to sixty hour weeks as I took over a legal case for another associate who had left the firm suddenly. Without any knowledge of her case, I was given less than two months to prepare for the trial and had to deal with intense filings, while preparing witnesses. At the time, a supervisor told me that the colleague I was going to trial with would, "celebrate you if you win the case, but put all the blame on you if you lose". The pressure felt immense.

On the day the trial ended (after successfully winning the case), I remember standing in the courtroom as my male colleague turned and walked out, leaving me to carry all the boxes by myself. It was incredibly symbolic of the fact that I was the one – literally – doing all the heavy lifting. It felt like he completely lacked empathy.

Even though I'd worked such long hours and successfully taken my former colleague's case to trial with the verdict being swung in our favor – whilst grieving the loss of my baby – I was still seen as 'damaged' and 'too emotional'. I'd really thought that my superiors would put me forward for partner, but instead, they promoted two of my male colleagues; neither of whom had gone to trial in the last few years, let alone recently.

I continued on with work, and in 2013, I fell pregnant again, and to our relief, we were blessed with a healthy child. However, as a result of my hours being 'down' after giving birth, I was once again held back from being promoted to partner. Whilst I was eventually promoted in 2014, I realized how much women were discriminated against in our workplace, and this was what led me to leave the firm several years later.

In hindsight, I now realize there were a lot of legal entitlements that I should have been offered after the loss of my child, yet none of these were mentioned. As an employment lawyer, it was probably assumed that I would know what options were available to me. But the truth is, the onus should not be on the employee to work this out. Employers should openly and enthusiastically supply their staff with this information, and say to them: "This is how much leave you currently have, and we encourage you to take as much as you would like or require during this time." It would have also been helpful to hear my employer tell me that lower hours due to pregnancy loss or having a child wouldn't result in retaliation or impact my chances of being made a partner.

To any supervisors, management teams, or workplace board members who may be reading this chapter, here are three pieces of advice I would like to share with you.

1. **Women who terminate their pregnancies need support, not judgment.** They need someone to spell out their rights clearly and to arrange for other team members to step in and support their workload, allowing them time to recover – both emotionally and physically. Workplaces need to ensure they have adequate systems and teams in place to support female employees when an unborn child is lost, as opposed to penalizing them for not making their hours or discriminating against that person for future career opportunities. Support needs to be enthusiastically offered. Don't wait for the female employee to ask for leave. In my experience, I was too scared to do so; scared of losing my job and worried about being seen as incompetent.

   As my husband noted to me while talking about sharing my story in this book: "When someone at work has a death in the family there isn't too much second-guessing about their need to drop what they're doing in order to be with their family. But it's not the same with an abortion – particularly one that is running up against the legal time deadline. How many places of work really have a safe and confidential means for employees to get access to their HR resources, be able to process that information, and then step away from work for however long is needed?"

2. **More needs to be done around workplace insurance and health options.** Though my policy covered some aspects of pregnancy, it did not include coverage for the screening tests that helped determine that my baby was facing critical health issues. Because these tests were deemed 'discretionary', I

ended up being thousands of dollars out of pocket and facing extreme financial hardship. Not only was this money that I didn't have at the time, but every time that rotten bill came in the mail, I burst into tears. I just didn't have the energy to advocate for myself or seek other support. If my insurance and health policy had covered these tests, it would have made the journey somewhat less traumatic.

It would also be great to see employers implementing a concierge-type health insurance service; a team who were there to help you navigate your options, and explain what might be covered by the insurance.

3. **Educational and anti-discrimination policies around miscarriage and late-term abortion are critical.** Particularly the latter. Although I am at peace with the decision I made for my child, I still grieve this loss more than nine years later. It was not an easy choice, and it caused immense emotional pain. It's important for workplaces and individuals in positions of power to understand the reasons that women seek out or have late-term abortions – and that, statistically, the numbers are much higher than what they likely expect.

There will be many female employees who have to consider a late termination for a child they desperately want, for no other reason than that it's in the best interest of the child or the mother. The truth is, we have more knowledge and resources than ever before to discover problems with babies before birth, but our medical system does not yet have the resources to save all of these babies.

Yet, due to the stigma attached to late-term abortions, many women do not speak up for fear of not just judgement, but also physical and verbal attacks from those who are anti-abortion. When female employees don't speak up, they are less likely to receive the support they need, and this can in turn negatively impact on their workplace (from a decrease in productivity, to an increase in absenteeism, and even the financial costs of having to replace an employee).

Though so much stigma still remains around experiences such as mine, I hope that by sharing my story I can help other women to advocate more effectively for themselves. And most importantly, that it will inspire workplaces and employers to look at how they can build healthier businesses where their female employees are supported, and not penalized for making the best decisions they can for their family.

TRISH - AUSTRALIA

I remember the moment I first discovered the lump. It was 2017 and I was sitting in bed watching television, preparing for a good night of sleep before my three-hour endurance run the next morning. For some reason my hand swept across my chest, and I felt a large, hardened lump on the left hand side. Given that it was quite high on the breastbone, I thought nothing of it. After all, I'd had a clear mammogram scan only six months prior, and no one in my family had a history of breast cancer.

I figured it was just a cyst that needed to be drained (a common experience for those of us with large breasts), so I pushed any concern out of my mind and went to sleep. The next morning, I completed my run in record time and enjoyed the rest of the weekend before getting ready for work on Monday.

That day, my hand passed over the lump again and I thought to myself: This is odd, but I really don't have time to go to the doctor. I'm sure everything will be fine.

The truth was, life was so busy at this time, as we were in the middle of a merger, and I had a team of twenty staff to manage and care for. Had I not (in passing) mentioned the lump to a female colleague – who immediately made an appointment for me, and essentially forced me to go to a local doctor in my tea break – then I would likely not have gone.

I'd barely had time to eat lunch and sit back down at my desk before my phone began to ring. It was the doctor – an urgent appointment had been scheduled for me the next day at the Wesley Hospital, and I needed to be there by 8am for testing. I advised my manager that I needed to take a day off for a medical appointment, to which he supportively encouraged me to "take as much time as needed".

Within twenty-four hours, I discovered that the lump was not a cyst as I'd thought – it was cancer.

Because of how serious the tumor was, I started treatment immediately, having a lumpectomy to remove the lump and doing twenty-four weeks of chemo followed by a two-week break and then six weeks of daily radiation. Everything happened so quickly, and it was a shock to someone like me who – in twenty-five years with the same organization – had rarely taken sick leave.

The impact on my body during my ten months of leave was enormous. Along with extreme fatigue, brain fog, and neuropathy in my hands and feet, I was also pushed into menopause as a result of the chemo.

In the beginning my team and management were very supportive, but as the months went by there was a lot of change within the management, and therefore I 'dropped off the radar' somewhat. While my immediate team were great and kept in contact regularly, my superiors weren't so proactive. It seemed as though they were more interested in who was going to take my role, to ensure the merger got through, as opposed to how to support me. Despite being extremely ill, I had to follow up with the pay office myself in order to arrange adequate sick leave and work out how to apply for additional leave from my super.

Due to the merger, everyone within management was made to reapply for their role, and this included myself. As I battled through chemo, I was told by a female manager that I would need to send through a resume and make myself available for a phone interview if I wanted a chance to retain my job as a team leader. After twenty-five years in the job, I couldn't believe I was being told to interview via phone. I've been with this organization for more than two decades. I'm a respected leader, I thought. In the end, they offered me an in-person meeting on a Friday at 3pm.

To give you some perspective, I had only just finished chemotherapy and was still undergoing radiation. To be asked to attend a meeting on a late Friday afternoon would probably be tiring for anyone, but when you're going through aggressive medical treatments, it's another thing entirely. In hindsight, I should have asked for a different time, but I didn't want them to think I was useless because I was sick. I felt I needed to prove myself.

As I stood in front of the mirror drawing on my eyebrows and fitting my wig into place, fatigue washed over me. I was so utterly exhausted, and I felt like I'd lost the battle for my job before I'd even entered the interview. "Good luck Trish, you're going to need it", was the advice given to me by a male manager as I walked toward the meeting room.

I could tell the panel had been stacked against me. They'd brought in two managers who had a history of not being very supportive of me or my leadership style, as well as an unknown HR manager from the merger. As I sat there in my itchy wig, sweating, and fighting for the role I had excelled in for so many years, I saw the visible discomfort on their faces as their eyes passed over my wig. The whole thing only made me more self-conscious.

Over the weeks that followed, I waited anxiously for an update. I'd asked one of my female managers how I would know if I'd been successful or not, and she'd assured me that I'd receive a phone call in the next few weeks to let me know.

"Don't worry Trish, we'll definitely let you know either way," she said.

Eventually the day came, and as I picked up the phone, my heart in my throat, I heard the words I'd been dreading: "Sorry Trish, you weren't successful in attaining the role." When I asked if she could share who the position was given to, I was advised that the company was still finalizing some details for the successful applicant and couldn't yet disclose the details – but not to worry, as I would receive a courtesy call to let me know very soon.

As it turned out, this never happened. Instead, I found out via text message weeks later from members of my team. It was only then that I discovered who my role had gone to.

I was offered a project role at the same level I was on, but it wasn't for me. Keen to make a difference and use my knowledge in more purposeful ways, I asked to be put into the billing team instead.

In the end, I was given a role as a billing officer; an admin position that was several levels below where I had been. Looking back, I should have fought harder, but I just didn't have the energy.

I stayed for around four months, after which time I was told that my role was no longer available, and my only options were to take a redundancy or accept a different admin position where my pay would drop by three levels.

I tried to go through our union, but I couldn't get any support, so in the end I took the redundancy.

Throughout my twenty-five years in this company, I'd always believed it to be the place I'd one day retire. I loved where I worked, and my mentors were amazing. Never did I ever imagine leaving the way I did.

There are so many things that my former workplace could have done to support me, and it all starts with leaders who understand emotional intelligence. It would have been hugely beneficial to have directors who checked in on me and how I was managing my recovery – both from a mental health and physical perspective. Often, I would get severe hot flushes from the chemo-induced menopause, but whenever I thought of taking my wig off in the office, I knew it would make others very uncomfortable. So, instead, I'd hide away in the toilet.

I also struggled with neuropathy in my hands and sitting behind the keyboard typing all day only made it worse. It was strange to see how passionate our workplace was about ergonomics and safety, yet no one encouraged me to take regular breaks, or looked into ways to balance my computer usage with non-digital tasks. Having a fan at my desk to assist with the hot flushes would have also been a small yet helpful gesture.

At no stage did I – or anyone in our team – know much about who was on the board of directors, other than to know that it was very male-dominated. We knew little about policies that were available, aside from who to talk to about ergonomic health and safety issues.

To this day, I still break down in tears when I think or speak about my experience. I took so much pride in my role, and for many decades I was an incredibly high performing employee with a huge team to care for and look after. Going through cancer and chemotherapy, along with the way I was treated when I returned, made me feel like everything had been taken away. Not only did my body betray me, but also my workplace.

Given that one in seven Australian women will face breast cancer in their lifetime (and those 2.3 million women were diagnosed globally in 2020 alone), it is so important for workplaces, management, and boards to understand that this is a disease that is likely to impact their staff at some stage. I would love to see workplaces and organizations partner with and receive training from breast cancer organizations and lived-experience advocates so that they can gain a better understanding of how to support survivors to successfully return to the workforce.

Above all, emotional intelligence, empathy, and awareness go a long way when it comes to creating a thriving and successful workforce.

JEAN – AUSTRALIA

"It's just 'women's problems.'"

As I lay on the floor of my classroom during recess, trying to sleep away the pain that seemed to rip through my body every month when my period hit, I thought about those four words. The pain was so unbearable that I found myself almost fainting, yet any time I tried to ask my doctor about it, they always said the same thing.

"It's just part of being a woman."

"Don't worry Jean, you'll grow out of it."

"You just need to eat more red meat. Get some additional sleep and you'll be right."

Unfortunately, it wasn't something I could grow out of, nor was it easily cured by diet. By the time I was twenty-three I was convinced there was something seriously wrong going on inside of my body. Sometimes, while driving, sharp pain would shoot through my vagina and into my back, almost like I was being electrocuted. Sex, too, had become incredibly painful.

Again, I was told that it was mostly just 'women's problems', but eventually, I was able to get a real diagnosis: endometriosis. The cysts and scarring were so severe, that it took a three-hour operation to remove them all. Unfortunately, I then developed an infection, which led to many other complications – particularly in my workplace.

Despite being in regular pain every month, I prided myself on being a productive employee, and doing what I needed to get through the day (Panadol, Panadeine, and heat packs were my go-to). Often, I'd be in incredible amounts of discomfort, yet I always did my best to paste on my 'work face' and manage the symptoms to the best of my ability. Sometimes this meant getting up from my desk multiple times per day to walk to the tearoom (helping to ease the back pain), or warm up a heat pack. To me, this didn't seem like an odd thing, but as I came to discover, it made my co-workers and management uncomfortable. Why? Because just the mere sight of a woman putting a heat pack on her lap made it very obvious that she was experiencing 'women's issues'.

Up until this point, I'd tried to be open with my co-workers when asked about endometriosis and why I needed to stand more regularly, or why I might not be as chirpy as everyone else. But their obvious discomfort only made me more self-conscious, which in turn, led me to believe that I shouldn't share what was going on with my health. It would have been so helpful to have a workplace that showed empathy or asked how they could support me, but instead, I was often on the receiving end of passive-aggressive comments and questions.

"Jean, is everything okay? You look like you have resting bitch-face."

"I know we all have issues going on, but you don't look very approachable. You need to make people feel more comfortable."

"You seem to take an awful lot of tea breaks Jean, is this something we need to talk about?" I wished that I could bring them inside my body for a day and show them what it was like trying to manage significant amounts of pain while also multitasking in a highly demanding role. It was like a full-time job on top of another full-time job.

"I just need to get up and move," I'd explain. "I get a lot of back pain and it's hard to sit down for ten hours at a time." "Yes, right. I see," they'd nod. Yet, it felt fake and judgmental.

I soldiered on, but in 2020, everything unraveled, and I found myself in more pain than I'd ever been in. I was working at a large company, handling the needs of multiple teams of accountants. Often, I worked twelve-hour days or even longer sometimes, and despite the agonizing pain I was often in, I gave my all. The fact that I had been able to function fairly well for many years was largely thanks to the fact that I had been fitted with a hormonal intrauterine device (IUD) – a small plastic T-shaped device containing progestogen, that is fitted into the uterus. However, it desperately needed to be replaced – otherwise I would become very ill, and risk not being able to continue working as I had been.

To try and avoid unnecessary disruption to my workplace, I explained to my employer that I would need a day off to have the procedure as I would be in a fair amount of discomfort afterwards and would therefore not be contactable for a specific period of time. Although I should have asked for additional time off, I didn't. Once again, that 'emotional obligation' to always be available was slapping me in the face. To my relief, my team seemed to understand, and all was well... or so I thought. I'd barely exited the doctor's office before my phone began vibrating with missed and incoming calls.

"Hey Jean, we just need your help to work this out."

"Hi Jean, can you tell me how to set this up?"

"Hey, just a quick question for you..."

Are you for real? I thought to myself. I'd given plenty of notice, I'd been super open about what I was going through, and I couldn't even get the afternoon off for medical treatment. Here I was high as a kite on prescription meds, and they still expected me to be working.

Shortly afterwards, I discovered that my endometriosis was so bad that I required urgent surgery. It ended up costing me more than $10,000. The real kicker was that, around this time, my workplace had pushed me to switch to a different health fund, telling me it was a far better option, and I should take it. Little did I know that this new fund would not cover me for my surgery.

So now, I was not only dealing with agonizing pain and stress around my upcoming surgery, but also the financial toll. Once again, I thought that if I was open with management about the procedure – when it would happen, and how much time I'd require off – that it would make it easier on the whole team. I explained to my female manager that the surgeons weren't sure how bad the endometriosis was, and that I may have stage-four scarring and cysts throughout my bowels. Unfortunately, they would have to explore to find out.

At this point, my manager stood back, her face awash with shock. "Fuck Jean, that's huge," she exhaled. "I didn't realize."

Even though I'd been talking very openly about my fears as well as the treatments I was facing, it wasn't until this moment that at least one of my managers understood just a little of what I was facing. After this conversation, one of my male managers approached and asked me to let him know if I needed any help. It sounded lovely, and he was saying all the right things, but I had a sense even then that his words felt performative and fake; like he was ticking a box.

This was confirmed to me in the days and weeks that followed. Not once was there a discussion from management as to how they could support me prior to, and after, surgery. There was no conversation about what tasks could be taken off my plate and given to someone else to reduce stress or assist me with recovery. Even when I shared openly with my team that I was burned out, nothing was done. "Okay, we'll look into it," is all that was said. No one seemed concerned about the fact that I was walking straight into Stage Four Endometriosis surgery off the back of a twelve-hour day.

On that day, as I lay in a hospital bed having just had extensive surgery, I looked down at my phone to see a message flash across the screen.

"Hey Jean, I need some help resetting my password. Can you help?"

I had not even been out of surgery for three hours. I felt so burdened to help, that I ended up doing it from my bed. This was a pattern and one that continued in the days afterwards. From 6am in the morning, I would be receiving text messages from one of our female managers about work, and even though I didn't report to her I felt obliged to respond.

In the end, I took only a week off work. In hindsight, I can see that I pushed myself so hard to come back early, when I should have been at home recovering. But I felt so much pressure to be there and show that I was capable. Unfortunately, nothing I did made any difference.

Within days of returning to work I was ordered – essentially – to attend a performance review. I remember asking if I could bring a support person with me, as I was in a fragile state following surgery, but this was not permitted. Although it felt incredibly odd to schedule something like this just after I'd had major surgery, I figured it would be a quick thirty-minute meeting and that I could get on with work and recovery. I was wrong.

For ninety minutes, I was barraged by the male director about how the 'team' didn't really like me and that I didn't fit in; that I wasn't 'approachable' or friendly enough.

I remember sitting there watching my recently operated on stomach swell larger and larger underneath my loose, post-surgery dress, as waves of nausea began to rise and a hot, burning feeling pulsed through my face. Panicking, I realized I had missed taking my post-surgery medication. The meeting had gone so long that I hadn't been able to get to my bag to take it, putting me at risk of illness or further infection.

In the moment, I just wanted to cry. How have I allowed myself to be treated this way? I thought silently. How did I get to this place where I am trying to please and put everyone else above my own health?

Unfortunately, as feared, I developed an infection a few days later, possibly contributed to by stress, but I guess I will never know. Yet even then, I was too afraid to talk to staff about what was going on. Quietly, I took myself to the Royal Women's Health Hospital, and on the way, texted the team manager to let them know where I was.

It wasn't until hours later that my male director messaged me to ask if I was okay. In a team of six people, it was obvious that I was missing, yet no one checked in. Because of the state of the infection, I needed a few days to recover and took a long weekend to try and get some rest so I could be back to work as quickly as possible.

During this time, I received a call from my director, saying there had been a 'meeting with HR' and it was vital that I be there. I tried to explain that I was away from work on sick leave, but this wasn't deemed an excuse. Given the pain I was in, and that my mind was still foggy from the surgery and recovery, I asked if I could bring a support person with me, but this was also denied.

To please them, I dialed in via telephone, where I was told that the reason an urgent HR meeting had been called was because I had 'snapped at a junior employee', and that I would now be issued with a 'formal, yet not formal' written warning.

Still hazy from the pain medication, I wracked my brain. Had I snapped at an employee? I couldn't remember doing so but given the enormous amounts of pain I'd been experiencing prior to, during, and after my surgery, it was possible that I may have unintentionally spoken harshly to someone.

When I explained this and apologized for any unintentional rudeness, the reply from my male manager was: "That's no excuse Jean. One of your KPIs is to be positive, remember? You're not meeting those standards, and we'll now have to issue with this written warning."

As I sat there on the phone trying not to cry, I was also advised very clearly that there would be no further career progression available to me in the next twelve months.

Within three weeks I left the company. To give you an indication of how quickly it all happened, I hadn't even had a follow-up with my surgeon. Yet in less than a month, I had effectively been forced out of my role.

It was devastating. I had worked twelve- to fourteen-hour days for this company and had always given my best. The worst part was that, had they allowed me more flexible working arrangements, I could have continued in my role. There are so many small things that could have been done, like having a conversation with me and coming up with an individualized plan instead of encouraging me 'not to talk about it'. Endometriosis is not just a woman's problem, it's a whole team issue – because when your staff aren't given adequate support to thrive, there is a negative flow-on effect to the rest of the department, as well as the company itself.

Having endometriosis is not just having a heavy period. It's not just something that women say to get time off work. It's very individualized to each woman, and like any disability, there are ways around it and things that you can do to make your staff feel valued and supported. Something as simple as putting sanitary products in the women's bathroom, so that when accidents happen you don't get stuck without supplies or have to try and awkwardly smuggle items into the toilets to avoid 'embarrassing' other staff, would go a long way. It doesn't have to be awkward.

You'll build a better workplace when you support women with endometriosis.

MELANIE – UNITED KINGDOM

My introduction to endometriosis began as a twelve-year-old girl. Even at that early age, I experienced agonizingly painful cramps and heavy bleeding, but like many young girls and women, I didn't know just how severe it truly was. There were occasions when my periods were so heavy, that I would literally have to wear a baby nappy to absorb the amount of blood being lost. After following up with a number of doctors I was put on the contraceptive pill around the age of fourteen, but that was the end of it. No one diagnosed endometriosis; they just noted that I had heavy periods which were impacting my iron levels and leaving me fatigued.

Understandably, the symptoms of endometriosis impacted me in many ways, particularly at school. On a physical level, I frequently felt lethargic and tired (likely due to insufficient iron levels) and I was also shy and uncomfortable about participating in sports. Growing up in the eighties, our gym uniform consisted of underwear/pants, and occasionally a short skirt – certainly not enough to hide a major bleed! As a result, I shied away from sports constantly. Nobody recognized the significant pain my periods were creating each month, nor the reason for my withdrawal from my peers.

I stayed on the contraceptive pill for three years until my periods became more regular and less heavy, yet even still, I was unable to achieve much on the first/second day of my cycle. This continued all the way through to my early thirties (when I finally achieved a proper diagnosis).

As an employee I rarely skipped work and was thankful that my career within the airline industry allowed me the freedom to work varied shifts/days. However, upon changing my career in my late twenties (moving into software and services), I experienced a lot of difficulties. Unlike my previous job, I was now in an office – and one which was very male dominated. Understandably, I never felt comfortable about opening up to my employer or team members about my pain, or the real reason for my sick days (which I took about once per quarter). Instead, I fell back on explanations of 'gastric issues' or 'food poisoning'. There was certainly nothing within our work policies that explicitly accommodated for menstruation issues or endometriosis, and similarly, there was zero education amongst management regarding support for staff who were struggling with such symptoms. This only encouraged me to keep my 'issues' to myself.

On one particular day, my stomach pains were so profound that I had to excuse myself in the middle of a meeting and head straight home. Some hours later, following a house visit by a doctor, I was in hospital. Only then were my symptoms finally given a formal name. Twenty years on from my first period, I was diagnosed with endometriosis.

After two decades, my body had created growths on both ovaries, one of which was four centimeters long (hence the incredible pain I'd been in!). Very swiftly I was taken in for surgery, and thankfully my ovaries were saved. However, even though the cysts had been removed successfully, there was uncertainty about my ability to have children should I decide to try and fall pregnant in the future. Returning to work, I found that my male boss was sympathetic but didn't want to know any details. It was a 'gynecological issue', and unlike other forms of surgery, there was an obvious reluctance to speak about it.

Whilst I'm thankful that endometriosis didn't impact my career in terms of advancement, I do believe that I often pushed my physical limits far more than I would now that there is much more understanding and discussion around this condition. At the time, I also felt that the medical profession was not well versed in methods of management of endometriosis – particularly given that I was taking the contraceptive pill for decades purely as a form of pain management, as opposed to a contraceptive measure (as a gay woman, the latter wasn't relevant to me).

Since entering menopause I've found that my condition now impacts me minimally. However, in my role as a Head of HR, I constantly strive to increase awareness of endometriosis, and the significant impact it – and similar female conditions – can have on the lives of women, including the challenge of getting pregnant. I also encourage and equip our management teams to better understand the mental health issues that can be experienced as a result, and the need to take additional time off to seek alternative treatments (including IVF).

I'm fortunate that the company I now work for is fairly open to recognizing female specific health matters such as menopause or endometriosis, and we drive frequent manager campaigns to help break down the reluctance to discuss such matters (which are simply a fact of life). Education and increased awareness of how menopause can impact performance is also a topic of priority on our agenda.

I'm grateful to have the opportunity to use my lived experience as well as my influence at work to continue making positive changes in this space. By sharing my story, my hope is that more people in positions of leadership will be inspired to deepen their understanding of what they need to do to create healthier, stronger, and more productive workplaces.

SONJA – UNITED KINGDOM

I experienced my first hot flash on my forty-sixth birthday. I distinctly remember it as though it were yesterday. I had taken myself out to a lovely cafe in Montreal, and while waiting for my breakfast to arrive, perched high on a stool, I felt a rush of heat unlike anything I had ever felt before. What the hell was that? I wondered. Like wildfire it spread throughout my body, forcing me to quickly begin shedding layers of clothing and dumping them on the ground beside me. I was sure, by now, that every other person in the room must have noticed the flaming human inferno in their midst, but not an eye was turned my way. As my brain whirred, I tried to make sense of what was happening. You have got to be kidding, that cannot be a hot flash, I thought, as I paused to catch my breath. I'm only forty-six.

Looking back, all the signs of what I now know to be perimenopause were there – including the subtle changes to my periods, which had begun to appear later, lighter, and some months not at all. It was during a visit to a friend who is a year older than I, that we got onto the subject of menopause. When I explained my symptoms, she told me I was definitely perimenopausal. Peri what? I thought.

As I began to research, I discovered that the average age of menopause is actually fifty-one, however in the many years preceding menopause, a woman goes through a transition phase called perimenopause – a period that, personally, I would compare to wandering in the wilderness while wondering, what the hell is going to happen to my body and mind next? The journey with menopause is not linear. For some it is passive and easeful. For others, including myself, it is like riding a rollercoaster that has no controls and you literally need to hang on tight and stay for the ride.

My experience, and my background in wellbeing, prompted me to begin uncovering the mystery of menopause and the often-unspoken misery of perimenopause and its impact on women. Why? Because no one talks about it! There is a lot of shame with ageing and entering the transition to menopause.

In my case, it wasn't until my forty-seventh birthday that I received an official confirmation. My gynecologist advised that my follicle-stimulating hormone (FSH) levels were declining, but not so low that I needed to consider hormone replacement therapy. I was happy with this advice, as my preference at this time was to do things 'the natural way'.

Around halfway through my forty-seventh year, I hit a real low with my perimenopause. I had returned to Australia, and my hot flashes were increasing in frequency, making it very difficult for me to teach. Often I would be in the middle of running a workshop or facilitating a class, only to be hit by rolling waves of hot flashes, which increased in temperature by the minute – like a person stoking a boiler inside me! I'd have to stop teaching or run to the bathroom to quickly peel off more layers of clothing and calm my mind.

During this time, I also noticed a steep decline in my mood. Instead of being my usual highly motivated and positive self, I began to feel agitated and anxious, with little motivation to do anything. At the time I had no idea what was going on and certainly didn't make any connection between my symptoms and menopause. I put the changes down to a busy schedule and life in general. I just didn't feel like me.

Desperate to understand what was happening, I went to see a local doctor – her advice was to consider antidepressants, which I declined.

"Come back in a few weeks if things don't improve," she suggested. I have no doubt her advice was given without any ill intention but was simply from a lack of understanding of the myriad of symptoms of perimenopause. That said, I left feeling lower than when I entered and went back to researching natural options.

From here, I also started to experience horrific night sweats. I would wake drenched to the core. It got to the point where I was sleeping naked with the window open during the middle of winter. As someone who runs cold, this was another 'what the fuck' moment.

The next year was absolute hell. Anxiety, low grade depression, brain fog, loss of confidence, headaches, nausea, poor sleep, and hot flashes all became regular features in my life. As you can imagine, the lack of sleep only exacerbated every single other symptom, and also led to a decline in my creativity and productivity. This was not ideal, as someone who was self-employed with a leadership and wellbeing business! During this time, I struggled to find the support I needed from the medical system because I wasn't really sure what I needed or who to ask, and this led to me feeling increasingly isolated and alone.

In early 2020 I returned to the U.K., just as the first wave of the pandemic hit. From here, things only worsened. My perimenopause was at its peak, and despite having severe anxiety and low-grade depression, I struggled on in silence. I didn't want to bother my doctor, as I didn't view it as an emergency and felt guilty at the thought of taking one of the limited appointments available when there were others out there who 'really needed it more than me'. The combination of COVID lockdowns and perimenopause led to a gradual yet increasing withdrawal from life, as I struggled on.

At this point, I had to make the difficult decision of pausing work as I was really struggling to function. For most of 2020 I struggled to work, and any projects I did undertake were pro bono to reduce stress and allow me to focus on my health.

I used the last of my savings and tried to figure out what to do next. It is only now, on reflection, that I can see how much I was struggling and how unwell I was. But in the middle of a crisis layered with a pandemic, it is really hard to move forward and get the help you need.

Over a period of three years, I had tried everything I could to manage my perimenopausal symptoms naturally. This including eating a clean vegetarian diet filled with green leafy veggies, using organic and natural supplements/powders designed for menopausal women, practicing daily yoga, meditation and breathing exercises, quitting alcohol and reducing caffeine, seeking psychological support, fasting intermittently, and using acupuncture. To an extent, each of these worked but not well enough. At this point, I knew I needed more long-term medical intervention.

At the age of forty-nine, I made the decision to start hormone replacement therapy (HRT). The tipping point came when my night sweats and itchy skin recommenced. I was pushed over the edge and needed help. Yet even so, it was not an easy decision for me to make, as I had convinced myself that HRT was not natural and not good for me. However, after a lot of research I came to the realization that my symptoms were not going to improve, and that in order to function fully and allow my brain and body to receive the estrogen and progesterone they needed, HRT was my only option.

Starting HRT felt like finding a doorway in a forest. I hadn't realized how much I had lost myself and my ability to function until I got back the hormones that had become so depleted. Finally, I had my life back. I only wish I had been supported to arrive at this decision sooner.

Right now, I am on a combined estrogen and progesterone patch. The oestrogen is identical to the type produced by my body, but the progesterone is synthetic (as the body-identical version is currently not available in Scotland; something I plan to seek advice from the government about as to why). Thankfully the hot flushes and night sweats have ceased, and my memory has returned (as has my zest for life, creativity and laughter). I am once again building my business and contributing to society.

During my journey, I was often given the option of antidepressants, but this was not what I needed. In reality, I knew that my body needed replacement of the hormones it was losing – particularly as oestrogen is so important to brain health. For every woman out there in the forty-five plus age bracket (and often younger), I would encourage you to regularly track your symptoms, as health professionals may not make the connection between what you are experiencing, and the correct treatment you need. Sometimes this can lead them to prescribe medication as the 'easiest' option – which may not be the right fit for you. In my opinion, our medical system is broken and needs a lot of work.

There is a global need to educate and change the conversation of menopause, to increase empathy and understanding, and to reduce the unnecessary suffering of millions of women and their loss from the workplace. Because the truth is, many women leave jobs that they love because of this natural evolution of being born female. They feel unsupported and unseen, and don't feel comfortable talking with their management teams. Further, many are discriminated against by their employers and fear losing their job – another reason why women often stay silent.

From working with other women who are navigating these changes, it is clear to me that there is little to no conversation between employers and their employees about the fact that society is impacted by menopause – not just women. There are few organisations with formal menopause policies, and whilst places like the U.K. are starting to change this through the uprising of a menopause revolution, we still have a long way to go.

Had I been working in an organization, I would have taken sick leave, but that would have required an understanding doctor, and not everyone understands menopause. Often, you get labelled as stressed, anxious, and depressed, but the underlying cause is the transition to menopause. I spent close to two decades in senior leadership in government and I have no memory at all of being given any information or training on how to support women in the workplace experiencing menopause. It just wasn't talked about.

By the year 2025, there will be one billion women experiencing menopause. Now is the time to destigmatize menopause, and increase education and accessibility to a range of treatments and support, because it's not 'one size fits all'. Businesses have an obligation to create policies that will support menopausal women, and boards need to have a diversity of gender and thought leadership to ensure an open and collaborative approach to menopause in the workplace, as well as ensure their policies are supportive and inclusive.

Menopause affects everyone. Women suffer, families suffer, relationships suffer, and the economy suffers. In fact, a 2019 report from HR Review UK highlighted that fourteen million workdays per annum were lost in the U.K. due to menopause. However, by normalizing conversations about menopause, a woman's employers, employees, friends, partner/husband, and children can better understand what is happening in her life, and how to be supportive.

There is a lot of wonderful work happening in raising awareness and education of menopause, but it is not yet enough. Menopause has been neglected by the medical establishment for decades and frankly, women have had enough. This is a personal journey for every woman, but it is time for businesses and governments to place women's health and menopause at the forefront of inclusive forward-thinking policies, to create cultures of belonging and wellbeing. It is time for a menopause revolution!

GENEVIEVE – AUSTRALIA

My first memory of living with dysmenorrhea (extremely painful menstruation), is an image of me curled up on the floor at age nineteen, as tears of agony streamed from my eyes and severe pain ripped through my body. It seemed so unfair to me that, as a woman, I had to suffer this torture every month – and I often wished that I could just wave a magic wand and become a man instead. As a young girl who loved gymnastics, I'd always been incredibly fit and agile, and didn't actually have a proper period until my late teens. However, once it arrived, it was debilitating and excruciating.

It wasn't until twenty-three that I received proper medical testing, at which point I discovered I had a small amount of endometriosis. I had a small laparoscopy, but as many women with endometriosis will know, surgery isn't a magical fix for many of the symptoms.

Just after graduating from university with a Bachelor of Visual Arts, I began working for a large security company that serviced a museum in Montréal, Canada. As an art student it was incredibly appealing, and I couldn't wait to spend my days working a meaningful job whilst being immersed in video art installations and contemporary paintings.

There was, however, one major issue with the job. Despite the long hours, we were not permitted to sit down during our shift – no matter the reason. As someone who took pride in my job, I had no issue with hard work, but it seemed strange that we weren't even allowed to sit for short periods of time to rest our feet. Over the past few years, I'd spent time travelling to many different cities in Europe, and had often seen security guards seated during the day for certain periods – so I couldn't understand the rigidity of the rules.

I remember the first time my period kicked in, after starting at the museum. Like every month, I was hit with a wave of dizziness and lethargy that was so severe that my legs would shake, and I'd feel as though I were going to faint. As the museum wasn't very busy, I decided to ask my manager – a thirty-five year-old man with a family of his own – if I could sit for a while, as I was concerned about fainting. His answer? Absolutely not.

For the first few months, I tried to hide my pain, gritting my teeth and pushing through. But on one particular day, I just couldn't take the cramping and tearing feelings any longer. At this point I'd been on my feet for about six hours, and I knew I couldn't last another minute more with the dysmenorrhea. "I'm so sorry, but I'm going to need to go home," I shared with my manager. "Would you be able to find someone to cover my last two hours?" He was livid, to say the least. To him, the fact that he had to pay a replacement security guard for a few additional hours was more upsetting than a staff member who was on the verge of fainting.

It was only a few weeks later that I was called into a meeting and advised that I was being transferred to another location. No longer would I be working in the beautiful museum filled with art I knew so much about – instead, I'd be put by myself in an empty, aged-care building. Every day I had to walk through a desolate twelve-storey high-rise that had previously been a hospital, making sure no one had broken in or vandalized it. In some ways, it was a blessing as I was able to sit or rest without being penalized, and although I was upset to have lost my dream job, being surrounded by creative people and art, I was relieved that I could at least rest during my period or bring a hot water bottle with me to work.

No reason was given for my transfer, but it was obvious that they found me too much trouble; a woman who spoke up too often and asked too many questions. Looking back, I should have contacted upper management, but as a twenty-four-year-old, I had little knowledge of my rights. I didn't even think to look at my contracts. On top of this, I felt like a troublemaker, always asking for permission or begging for simple human rights.

A few months later I was moved again, this time to this time to the famous McGill underground tunnel area in the Westend of Montréal, as upmarket shops needed security. It was a much better environment where I was able to sit or rest when needed, and one that was definitely more exciting. Sometimes my days were spent chasing after, tackling and catching thieves. It felt good to be in a job where I was needed and could utilize my skills. Yet, at the same time, I still in a male-dominated industry where there was zero talk about what our rights were, or what policies were available for health issues.

One of the biggest issues for women in the workplace is the fact that so many people in positions of leadership still fail to understand the impact that issues like dysmenorrhea, endometriosis, and other female-only health conditions have on women. In my experience, my career has absolutely been impacted by each of them, and they have severely affected my ability to maintain a job.

Every woman has different experiences when it comes to menstruation, yet there's little support when it comes to things like dysmenorrhea. This is one of the many reasons that I ended up working for myself – simply so that I wouldn't have to answer to management about the pain I experienced monthly. However, even now, as the head of a not-for-profit organization, I have still experienced many difficulties in the last ten years as a result of my biology. At times I have been so weak from pain, that it has been difficult to get into the office. This, coupled with pregnancy, giving birth to three children, and having to continue working throughout with little support, has made it very difficult to continue my career.

Although I'm currently going through early menopause (a genetic condition that also affected my mother), I think it's important to note that I had twenty years of severe pain prior to now. Is it any wonder so many women leave the workforce early, or retire with little to no financial security?

To any leaders, CEOs, or management who are reading this book, I would like to share this: The rigidity around rules 'in the office' really needs to be shifted. Workplaces talk about diversity – but they aren't considering diversity when it comes to supporting female staff. We see many supervisors and leaders who are happy to provide additional leave or flexibility for employees of particular religions/faiths (such as creating prayer rooms within the office building to allow Muslim employees to take breaks during the day for their required prayer times), so why are women still fighting to be given basic employee flexibility/support for biological functions that impact them every month?

Menstruation and female biological health issues impact half our population, and they don't need to be stigmatized. Nor, do they mean that women aren't committed to their jobs, or that they're incapable of thriving in their role. I promise you this: Your workplace will be happier, stronger, more productive and profitable when you improve inclusivity and support options for women in the workplace.

The Role of Culture

When considering the issue of women's equality, one of the things that cannot be underestimated is the role that culture plays. People often fail to recognize the significant differences that exist from one culture to the next and how this impacts employees, managers, and organizations. In my role as an international lawyer, I see this frequently in a number of areas of my work. When managers are responsible for staff in other countries it can often present cross-border challenges. The laws vary significantly from one country to the next, but it is a lot more complex issue than just differences in the law. Cultural norms, beliefs and values impact the way in which we manage conflicts and other situations in our personal and professional lives. For global organizations with teams that work together across borders, this can prove challenging to manage.

One of the areas of practice I have had a lot of experience in, is with assisting clients to manage global complaints and investigations. Throughout my eighteen years of legal practice, I have run hundreds of investigations, and, because of my international focus, many have involved complainants and witnesses across multiple countries. One issue I have seen many times in investigations is a lack of appreciation and understanding for the differences in the culture, beliefs, values, standards, and laws of one country to the next. I have seen employees express frustration over various issues that have occurred because their managers have failed to understand or respect their differences and I have equally seen managers express frustrations for similar reasons.

I will always remember a client who sent an executive from South Africa to manage a team of employees in Japan and Australia. Because the client had not undertaken to train the executive on some of these cultural and country-specific issues, the executive was unable to manage an effective team. Employees ended up going off work on stress leave. Several employee complaints were made and productivity within the business plummeted. As I interviewed the various parties to the dispute, including the executive, it became clear to me that the executive was not acting as a result of any ill-intent or malice, but rather it was directly a result of a lack of understanding of these issues. The executive was simply acting and managing the team as he had always done – as he knew how to do effectively within his country of birth, where he had lived and worked his entire career. He had been asked to relocate to manage the team in Australia and Japan as a result of his proven track record in turning around other failing parts of the business. However, his management style simply did not work when placed in these two very different countries. He was viewed as aggressive, unreasonable and his style almost militant. The employees did not understand or respect his approach because they did not personally feel valued, understood or supported by the manager. This led to a situation of chaos, which was the point at which I was asked to step in and assist.

This is not an isolated example by any means. I see these types of issues arise frequently when advising U.S. headquartered companies about termination laws in Australia and New Zealand. I am often confronted with perplexed clients when I explain that there is no concept of 'at-will' employment in most countries outside of the U.S. and, in fact, not only does there need to be a valid reason for the dismissal, but a procedurally fair process must be followed and the concept of natural justice adhered to in many countries as well.

When I am asked to assist, it is often at the point where various steps have already been taken, an employee threatens a lawsuit for failure to adhere to the law or the former employee has already filed a claim. In both of these scenarios, once I review the facts I am often left with similar conclusions as I am during my involvement in investigations. Culture, values and local laws are sometimes overlooked and it is assumed by the person or team that is handling the matter – and addressing the issue in line with what they know and therefore understand – that it is the correct approach. Despite this, it often results in legal and sometimes reputational risk as well.

Another area where I see this arise regularly is in respect to client requests to implement global policies, or policies that are consistent across multiple jurisdictions – a task that is simply not possible in many cases and once again all of the issues outlined above come into play. Additionally, while employees in the U.S. may prioritize compensation for example, employees in Europe may care more about the leave entitlements and retirement benefits that are being offered by an organization. Market rate standards on many of these aspects of the employment relationship vary widely from one part of the world to another. These are considerations that organizations will need to factor into their decision making around how best to balance the desire for consistency across an organization globally and meeting the needs of their local workforce, while remaining legally compliant. It is also an equally important consideration as companies attempt to grow teams within new countries by head-hunting top talent to join what is often a new player in the local market.

It is worth noting that I generally see most mistakes made in situations where it involves people from one English-speaking country to another – for example, the U.S and Australia. In my view, the reason for this is that we are tricked into a false belief that our common language makes us similar. For example, as Australians we grow up in a society that is very influenced by the U.S. culture and so much so that we are almost tricked into believing that as a country and society we are very similar to the U.S. After living and working in the U.S. for over ten years, I can tell you with some certainty how far from reality that belief actually is. Although we speak similarly, we do not speak the same language at all. We are culturally very different. While there are some lifestyle similarities between the two countries, the differences are greater and the laws vary widely, not least because the U.S. legal system provides such a broad contrast from one state to the next, whereas Australia's laws often apply at a federal level in many areas and where they do not, the differences are typically minimal. This is just one example, but the same degree of variance applies between New Zealand and Scotland or Canada and Ireland. Factoring in even the small differences that may seem insignificant can mean the difference between success and failure in a new market.

I will never forget early on in my career in the U.S. when I drafted a document for a client's Australian office with Australian spelling, only to receive an email from the client after they had reviewed my work to complain that the document was full of spelling errors. I learnt a simple lesson early on that we should never assume another person is aware of these types of differences. I am grateful that client provided me with the opportunity to explain, but under different circumstances I could easily have lost a client that just assumed I was sloppy and failed to use spellcheck on my work before providing them with the final product. That experience, and many others like it since, have demonstrated to me time and again just how crucial it is to understand the market in which you are operating, and the various nuances that exist from one to the next. Needless to say, I now always explain these types of differences to new clients when working with them for the first time. Equally, employers also need to take the time to explain these types of nuances to their managers, who are managing employees across borders.

It is because I see first-hand the types of issues that can arise as a result of failing to adequately consider culture that I regularly advise companies to invest adequate resources and time in properly training, coaching and implementing support mechanisms for managers and executives to effectively and successfully manage their global teams. Companies should be impressing upon their leadership the importance of learning about and taking the time to understand the cultural and legal differences of a new market and its people. It is important to manage legal risk and ensure good corporate governance and compliance, but there are other reasons why this is important as well.

So, that brings me back to the issue. You might now be asking what this all has to do with women's health issues and the workplace. Well, what we know is that the global statistics on workplace equality do look markedly different from one part of the world to the next. Take for example the number of women in the workplace in China, which is forty-eight percent, yet women in CEO roles sits at about twenty percent, and women on boards at about nine percent. In the U.S., although women hold almost fifty-two percent of management and professional level jobs is the U.S., women lag significantly behind men when it comes to holding leadership roles.

For example, in 2021 women only hold 22.7 percent of all partner positions in law firms, sixteen percent of medical school deans and 15.5 percent of chief financial officer positions. In Australia, women constitute forty-two percent of the workforce but only hold twenty-five percent of executive positions and only ten percent of CEO positions in large, for-profit companies. The percentage of women on boards sits at just eight percent in Japan compared to 35.4 percent in the U.K. and less than thirty percent in New Zealand. The percentage of women in the workforce in France is 48.13 and women hold 29.7 percent of board positions versus South Africa, where women make up 45.47 percent of the workforce and hold 20.7 percent of board roles.

Part of the reason for the variance between countries relates directly back to culture and the long histories of countries, their people, beliefs, traditions and views. Expectations about the traditional behaviors and roles of men and women and about the relations between both sexes are fundamental aspects of culture and they shape daily life – personal and professional. As many more men went to work while women stayed at home in traditional homemaker roles, it is unsurprising that the workplace was largely built by men for men, but as we know, things are changing globally.

It is also important to recognize that the pace of change can be, and often is, quite different from one part of the world to the next. As I am writing this chapter of the book, the situation in Afghanistan with the Taliban overthrowing the government and taking control of the country has just happened. This is an extreme example of the persecution of women at its worst and the rolling back of years of progress for women's rights, but it is nonetheless a very real example that is still relevant today.

In China, there has been a decline in female participation in the workforce since the 1990s, which many contribute to the gender stereotypes that still remain as women continue to be seen as the primary caregivers and are expected to stop work to care for their families. There are also other examples that we see frequently in more progressive countries such as Australia and the U.S. where women continue to be subjected to sexual harassment, discrimination, and disadvantage in workplaces in alarming numbers. And what is the answer? How can we hope to really effect significant change if so many of the challenges that women face in the workplace and in life generally relate back to a country, its people and the culture? Well, it starts with education, changing the narrative within our own homes and our own communities and by living by example for our children and others around us. This is also another reason why mentors and sponsors are so important as I discuss more in **The Importance of Mentors and Sponsors.**_

Change can also happen when enough people publicly demand it, but as we are all creatures of habit, change can be difficult. This is not, however, an excuse for us not to continue to try. We have seen many examples over recent days around issues regarding race in the U.S. and other parts of the world, but as we have seen in Japan, South Korea, China, Indonesia, and India, which are all countries that have implemented period leave laws that are not widely utilized, cultural issues often stand in the way of women accessing the benefit[44].

Interestingly, Japan implemented period leave more than seventy years ago after World War II and initially there was a relatively high take-up of approximately twenty-six percent, but usage has significantly dwindled since, with less than one percent now estimated to access the benefit. One of the reasons for this could be that while the law mandates the leave, there is no obligation on employers to pay for the time off work and many companies do not promote that the leave is available to their employees. Women in many Asian countries also face some of the highest gender pay gaps in the world, so it is unsurprising that they would not be keen to access a benefit that could generate a negative response. In contrast, Zomato, a food delivery company in India, is encouraging its employees to access period leave when needed and attempting to break down the stigma attached to the issue. As Deepa Narayan, a social scientist and former senior adviser at the World Bank says, "The problem is work, not women".[45]

---

44. https://www.cnn.com/2020/11/20/business/period-leave-asia-intl-hnk-dst/index.html

45. https://www.cnn.com/2020/11/20/business/period-leave-asia-intl-hnk-dst/index.html

In Australia, the 2020–21 Leave for Loss campaign initiated by the Pink Elephants Network[46] provides us with a great example of when public campaigning on an issue does work. In this example, and many others, where a movement has triggered significant change, there are always those who will push back and oppose the change, because change to culture and values has implications for everyone. It also often results in changes to the law, which is ultimately what we need to see for widespread improvements in gender equality globally.

The Pink Elephants Network underwent a public campaign to drive support from members of the public and businesses, many of whom got behind the campaign in support of changes to the law to provide for paid leave entitlements for miscarriage. At Megaport, when we learned of the campaign we immediately wanted to get on board. Rather than simply wait for changes to be legislated by the government, instead we chose to be proactive and introduced paid leave for all of our employees globally – in situations where they or their loved one suffered a miscarriage. Many other companies also made similar decisions to move ahead of the law and implement miscarriage benefits. By doing so, it starts to create a ripple effect towards change. When governments can see that there is real public support behind an issue, they will usually take notice. This is how we change culture. By making changes within organizations and encouraging others to follow suit, this fosters a societal change in the culture of industries, communities and eventually, more widely within cities, states, or countries. This is another reason why I believe that every single organization has a role to play in moving the needle closer toward achieving gender equality.

Another area where I see employers playing a key role in workplace gender diversity is in the area of parental leave. Unfortunately, the number of men that take parental leave remains relatively small globally. One reason for this is that so many companies still adopt an age-old distinction between 'primary' and 'secondary carer'. I am pleased to say that we eliminated this distinction within the organizations that I am a part of, but while the

---

46. https://www.pinkelephants.org.au/

number of countries where paternity leave has now been introduced in law has doubled in the last twenty years, globally, only one in ten organizations provide paid paternity leave[47]. Another issue is the fear of negative repercussion on career prospects that remains. "Gender stereotypes are not only descriptive but also prescriptive. They can be quite damaging and limiting as they create a narrative of what the roles and prioritizes of both men and women should be.

Age and generations within culture also impact views around many of these issues. There is evidence to suggest that younger generations are much more accepting of health issues being workplace issues that employers need to address and support, and they are demanding change more than past generations. Older workers often have the opposite view and many feel that because they struggled through work while dealing with their own health issues, younger women should do the same.

I have been faced with older female family members who have expressed the same views to me, and my answer is always the same: "You're right. However, how many women were in management, executive or board-level positions in your day at work? And what was equality in the workplace like back then? Or the pay gap back then between men and women? We want change because we want equality and that cannot happen without finding better ways to support women at work." That type of response usually gets opponents thinking about the issue a bit differently. You might like to try it, too.

Of course, we must be respectful and sensitive to every culture, country and its people and their beliefs. However, respect is not the same as acceptance and a respectful way of influencing change is through education, consultation, and discussion. Rome wasn't built in a day, but someone had to lay that first brick.

---

47. https://www.bbc.com/worklife/article/20210712-paternity-leave-the-hidden-barriers-keeping-men-at-work

Why We Need More Women on Boards

Diversity on boards is critical to performance. It is not just nice to have, it is something that has been proven time and again to directly impact an organization's performance and profitability. Yet diversity on boards is something that remains largely under-valued.

In 2012, Italy introduced a law that requires public and state-owned companies to have at least one-third female board members by 2016. The law was introduced as Italy had one of the lowest female board member participation rates on the planet. In 2021, California introduced similar requirements under SB 826, California's board gender diversity law. The law requires that publicly held companies (defined as corporations listed on major U.S. stock exchanges) with principal executive offices located in California, *no matter where they are incorporated*, include minimum numbers of women on their boards of directors. Under the law, each of these publicly held companies was required to have a minimum of one woman on its board of directors by the close of 2019. That minimum increases to two by December 31, 2021, if the corporation has five directors, and to three women directors if the corporation has six or more directors. The legislation also authorizes the imposition of fines for violations of the law in the amounts of $100,000 for the first violation, and $300,000 for each subsequent violation.

These laws seem to have had the desired effect, with a report from the California Partners Project[48] showing that as of late 2020, less than three percent of public companies with principal offices in California remain with all-male board members. It is unfortunate that we need law makers to impose gender diversity requirements

---

48. https://www.calpartnersproject.org/claimyourseat2020

on boards, but if this is what is it going to take to improve board diversity, then we need more countries and states to follow suit.

There are many benefits to appointing women to boards. A 2015 McKinsey report on public companies found that those in the top quartile for gender diversity were fifteen percent more likely to achieve better financial returns than their competitors in the industry. Numerous studies show that companies with female board members generally see competitive advantages in terms of higher net margins, higher profitability, and lower share price volatility. Many experts also believe that companies with female directors also tend to manage risk more effectively, because they tend to look at issues by focusing on a wider perspective when considering the interests of their shareholders, employees, customers, the industry and the community.

There are other important reasons why having women on boards makes good business sense. Women represent the largest market opportunity in the world. Globally, women control or influence over $31.8 trillion in annual consumer spending or eighty-five percent! When you think about how staggering this number is, it is amazing more companies don't appreciate that women as consumers would make great board members given that they account for so much of the decision-making around spending. Of course, the numbers do vary from one industry to the next, but if we look at an industry such as the beauty industry, it is still amazing that it remains an industry that is dominated so heavily by men, yet overwhelmingly targets women.

As of March 2021, women hold only fifteen percent of CEO positions in the top twenty beauty manufacturing companies globally. This compares to the even worse statistic though of just forty-one female chief executives or 8.1 percent of the Fortune 500[49]. The figures are even more dismal for women of color with only two Black women running Fortune 500 companies. These figures actually represent an improvement from prior years, but demonstrate just how far we still have to go.

---

49. https://fortune.com/2021/06/02/female-ceos-fortune-500-2021-women-ceo-list-roz-brewer-walgreens-karen-lynch-cvs-thasunda-brown-duckett-tiaa/

Women who sit in executive and board-level roles also serve as role models for other women within organizations and they demonstrate that those positions are possible for other women within their organization and, more broadly, in the community. Research shows women leaders are more likely than male leaders to speak publicly about gender and racial equality at work[50]. If we don't see other women in these types of roles, younger generations are far less likely to strive for those positions because they view them as unattainable for people like them.

This is also representative of the importance of diversity within organizations generally. Minority employees need role models and examples of others who have achieved success so that they too can develop similar goals to strive towards. If a person of color only sees white employees at the top, their motivation to strive towards those positions is likely to be limited. And we desperately need more diversity at the top to provide different perspectives on how to work towards better workplace equality.

Black women have always experienced greater difficulties and barriers at work. They are promoted less, it takes longer to be awarded a promotion, and they are significantly underrepresented in management, executive and board-level roles, which means there are fewer opportunities for other women of color coming up through the ranks to connect with more senior leaders. Research has also shown us that Black women have suffered the affected of COVID-19 disproportionally. Now more than ever, the workplace needs to be a safe and supportive environment for all women, especially women of color.

If we continue to have conversations about diversity with boards and leadership teams that all look the same, yet expect different results, we are kidding ourselves. Just as I would not presume to understand what it is like for someone who is autistic or dyslexic in a workplace environment, so too do I expect the organizations I work with to listen to people like me when it comes to issues impacting women with fertility struggles and health issues such as endometriosis, and our experiences in the workplace. If an organization seeks the

---

50. https://www.mckinsey.com/featured-insights/diversity-and-inclusion/women-in-the-workplace#

advice of men within the organization and leaves up to those men its decision-making about the conditions, benefits and support that women in similar circumstances need, how can they possibly expect to be able to create a workplace environment of equality where men and women are provided with equal opportunities? It is laughable. Yet, these types of discussions occur every single day within organizations, on boards and in governments that are heavily male dominated. The idea that men will assume they know the needs of women is not a new concept, it is just an entirely outdated one.

If we look at the health care industry for example, the statistics on medical clinical testing and research can be frightening. Gender bias in medicine and medical research has caused significant risk to women's health issues for centuries, with women often taking significantly longer to be diagnosed with conditions that impact both genders. Why? Well, it relates directly to historical medical research and clinical testing. Women were often excluded from medical research and testing.

In 1977 the US Food and Drug Administration (FDA) recommended women of childbearing age be excluded from clinical research studies. Women have also been excluded from clinical trials because a woman's menstrual cycle causes hormone variations, which can affect results. This variable means that using women in trials can extend the testing and, in turn, increase costs. Because of this, women were often excluded, and it was assumed that whatever was safe for men would have similar results for women. This has turned out to be a false assumption many times over with drugs having to be withdrawn for use as a result, with higher percentages of women suffering adverse side effects over the years due to a lack of sufficient testing. Unfortunately, though, the issue is one that is still present, even today. According to the latest figures from the Australia Talks National Survey 2021[51], more than one in three women say that they have had health concerns dismissed by a doctor[52].

---

51. https://australiatalks.abc.net.au/

52. https://www.abc.net.au/news/2021-06-07/women-health-concerns-dismissed-gender-gap-australia-talks/;

Studies have shown us that the presence of women is necessary to change the culture and dynamics of a board and even more broadly within an organization. Women have lived experiences as women in the workplace. They are therefore best placed to develop and drive strategy that assists to attract, retain, and support other women to succeed. Diversity on boards doesn't matter much though, where board members' perspectives are not listened to and valued.

To make diverse boards effective, the board needs to develop and foster a culture of inclusion where board members are encouraged to voice ideas and express opinions and where those ideas and opinions are genuinely considered. This is critical to change the gender imbalance in industries that are male dominated, such as mining and construction, agriculture, finance and even the tech industry. To make it easier for women to enter into these types of industries, remain and succeed, we need women at both board levels and in executive and management roles – women who are in positions of power with the ability to influence the culture of an organization and its people, and women who have a voice and a seat at the table to assist in the development of strategies within the organization.

The board chair and lead director also have the responsibility to step up and ensure that the other board members have opportunities to voice opinions or ideas in a respectful manner. Friendly debate is healthy, and it is essential for the effective operation of any board – but shutting down ideas that we may not agree with, without providing a person with an adequate opportunity to share those ideas, is disrespectful and undermines the roles and responsibilities of each board member. Board chairs typically set the tone for the operation and effectiveness of the board and each of its members, so it is important for organizations to consider this when looking to appoint a person to such an important role.

The current push for social change with the introduction of the #MeToo movement, Black Lives Matter and similar social movements that have followed around the world, has sparked consumers, investors and even job candidates to start asking questions about an organization's diversity profile and strategy, and ultimately more is being demanded of organizations in these areas. Clients now want to know about the composition of the board and the workforce, what the diversity goals of the organization are, what benefits and opportunities are provided to women and minority employees and what the organization's strategies are for improving its diversity profile. Many investors have more of a social conscience today, with many now doing their research to determine the culture and values of an organization before deciding whether to place their investment there.

Many traditional and conservative industries, such as pensions funds and investment banks, are also increasingly being asked to explain why they do not have more women on their boards and what their strategy is for future change. Customers are finally starting to demand change, and this is something that every single one of us should be doing every day through the consumer choices we make – from purchasing groceries right through to major purchases such as a car or property. Take time to think about the organizations you are supporting through your purchases and, where possible, seek out organizations that have clear public diversity and inclusion strategies, companies that are run by female CEOs or those that have a strong female presence and those that clearly prioritize diversity.

With an increasing focus on diversity and inclusion, it is really not difficult to seek out organizations with a clear approach to improving opportunities for their women and minority workers. We live in an age of technology and every day it is becoming easier to gather this kind of information about companies. If a brand that you love is silent on these issues, it probably means they do not view diversity and inclusion as a priority and, in my opinion, they are the organizations to try and avoid.

The fact is that having an even balance of men and women within your organization and women on your board is good for the organization's bottom line and studies have consistently shown this. Yet the percentage of women on boards has barely increased globally in over a decade even though women earn fifty-seven percent of bachelor's degrees, over sixty-two percent of master's degrees, and fifty-three percent of degrees such as PhDs, medical degrees, and law degrees in the United States[53]. One area where the statistics have improved though is in ASX public company boards in Australia. In August 2021, for the first time in history, there were no all-male boards on any of Australia's top 200 companies[54].

Having women, and in fact more diversity on your board generally, broadens your contact base and talent pool. Hiring more women is important at all levels, but placing a woman on a board can set the tone for the organization and makes a statement about the organization's diversity objectives. I have certainly experienced this myself, as I was the first woman appointed to one of the boards that I serve on. Since joining the board, I can think of numerous situations where I have encouraged the organization to consider appointing a female candidate for many reasons. In turn, this has assisted us to move the needle towards a more balanced male-female ratio and a more diverse workforce, and the results speak for themselves. We have seen many positive changes within our teams and our organization as a result. The fact is that if you want to build an organization that is capable of innovation, you need diversity in your teams.

It is not only important for women to see examples of other women at the top of their organization, but as women make up approximately 46.9 percent of the workforce globally, having women on the board also means that an organization's employee population is more accurately represented. The Women's Leadership Foundation[55] released a report titled *The Value of Women on Boards of Directors – Looking Beyond Results*[56] and the report outlines some of the top reasons why women improve corporate performance on boards, including the following, which I leave you with as some additional food for thought:

- Women tend to use logic and facts in addressing positions held by those with dominant opinions
- Women tend to be inclusive and inviting of the thoughts and opinions of others

53. https://www.hsph.harvard.edu/ecpe/why-diversity-matters-women-on-boards-of-directors/

54. https://www.moneymag.com.au/no-all-male-boards-asx-200

55. https://womensleadershipfoundation.org/why-women-on-boards

56. https://womensleadershipfoundation.org/s/WLF-The-Value-of-Women-on-Boards-Beyond-Results-June-2018-B0D0A-Heck-lbdc.pdf

- Women often seek ways to challenge effectively
- Multiple studies show that women are adept at fostering strategy development, improving corporate social responsibility related issues and are highly effective in monitoring management
- Women's presence on boards can contribute to cohesiveness
- Studies show that women spend more time preparing for board meetings, have better attendance records than men, and improve the attendance behavior of male board members
- Women tend to have a significant positive effect on board development activities such as board instructions and board evaluation
- Women often champion difficult or controversial issues and help broaden discussions to better represent the concerns of a wider range of employees
- Women can contribute to the creativity or innovation of board discussions and of solutions to issues that are discussed and considered at a board level

Tackling the Opposition

During the time that I have spoken out about issues impacting women in the workplace, I have repeatedly heard the following reasons why some people are opposed to workplace change in the area of women's health:

1. This is all great, but I am trying to run a business and make money/these types of initiatives would cost too much.
2. Women have a hard enough time in the workplace without highlighting our differences.
3. I don't want my employer knowing about my personal health issues.
4. Health issues are not a workplace issue.

I understand that each of these things are very different, but also very real concerns for some people. For this reason, I want to tackle the opposition for you now. My hope is that for those of you that are not yet convinced, that you might start thinking about this issue in a different way by analyzing some of the data. Those of you that are already believers, I hope that this chapter might give you some useful arguments to use next time you are confronted with opposition around issues impacting women at work.

COST VERSUS PROFIT & PRODUCTIVITY

So, let's begin with the issue of cost and the link between wellness, profit, and productivity. Most organizations are in the business of making money, or if they are not, then they at least have a vested interest in getting the best productivity out of an employee to achieve certain results. That is completely reasonable and obviously to be expected. After all, why else do people run businesses unless they are not-for-profit organizations with a charitable cause? I also do not want to give the impression that I think hard work is a bad thing. Indeed, it is the opposite. Like everything in life, if we demonstrate hard work, focus and commitment, then we are much more likely to generate positive results.

When asking for help, support, or resources, you are more likely to get a favorable outcome when you are coming in from a position where you have a proven track record of performance. Not only is your employer a lot more likely to want to support you so that they can retain your talent, but it also arms you with arguments as to why providing you with that support is not only going to assist you to succeed, but it makes sense for the business as well. Unfortunately though, employee health and wellness is not a priority that has been traditionally integrated into the culture and corporate goals of many organizations.

Most companies do recognize that there is a cost to losing staff, but the costs are often more significant than realized. There are numerous studies that show the cost of an employee's resignation can range from thousands of dollars right through to two times the employee's annual salary. If a person leaves, the organization must spend time and resources on recruitment efforts which can take weeks or even months in some cases, but there are often also additional hidden costs to the recruitment process.

When an employee resigns and an alternative candidate is eventually found, there is an onboarding process and period of training or handover. There are very few jobs where a person can start today and immediately hit the ground running. Most people need some guidance and induction into the role and the systems and policies of an organization before they can perform the job effectively without assistance. In some cases, this can take weeks or even months. Additionally, there are cost savings to be had where your existing employees refer others in their networks for open roles, but naturally this will generally only occur where an employee is satisfied in their employment.

Therefore, the true cost of an employee resigning far outweigh merely the cost of recruitment and can include lost productivity and lost engagement, as well as impacts of team culture and performance. Employees also become more valuable over time. Existing employees have knowledge of the business and its functions, and knowledge of the requirements of their position. This is valuable and sometimes it doesn't hurt to remind an employer of this because, in my experience, it is something that is often undervalued. Employees are replaceable in most cases, but replacement does take time, money and resources which is something that should be factored into any consideration.

There are many other benefits that flow on as a result of providing better support for women at work, many of which may directly or indirectly affect the bottom line of the business. When employees feel well and healthy, they are more focused, have more energy and are more productive. The reality is that wellness programs and investing in employee wellness more broadly is frequently linked with qualitative outcomes such as improved employee morale, engagement, job satisfaction, reduced absenteeism, and reduced stress.

Supporting people when they are unwell, also assists them to return to work in a healthy state which leads to improved productivity more quickly. 'Value on investment' has become a method used by some companies to evaluate the effectiveness of wellness initiatives and programs by looking at the broader financial impacts that these programs, as well as employee benefits and policies, can have on an organization.

This method of evaluation looks at medical cost savings, reduced absenteeism, employee satisfaction and engagement, productivity, reduced turnover, improved rates of retention, reduced recruitment costs and increased innovation. Businesses that only consider one of these things when evaluating wellness initiatives really are missing out on the big picture of how valuable and effective these initiatives really are. Having employee benefits that are not utilized heavily, does not necessarily mean that they are not effective or valued by employees. Employee paid miscarriage benefits are a good example of this. Obviously, we hope that employees do not experience a miscarriage and need to access the leave. However, merely knowing that it is there should they suffer a miscarriage carries enormous psychological benefits. One of the best ways to evaluate wellness initiatives, policies and benefits is to ask your employees directly through surveys, group think-tank sessions or other forums, where employees are provided with opportunities to share their thoughts, ideas, and feedback for improvements.

An organization's employee wellness strategies also link directly to its employment brand and public image. As employees and job candidates are demanding more from companies in relation to health and wellness, gone are the days where a focus on employee wellness is a 'nice-to-have'. Rather, all companies should now be adopting a culture of wellness as a default if they want to attract and retain good talent. Clients, too, are increasingly looking to work with service providers that are more aligned to their own values and culture. RFIs often ask for a company's diversity profile and for information about diversity and inclusion initiatives and employee benefits. As technology becomes more and more advanced every day, our visibility into these things also continues to improve. No longer can companies hide away or simply stay silent without assumptions being drawn about their priories on these issues.

Recruitment firms and companies that offer employee engagement and people management solutions often conduct useful research into issues around employee benefits, including wellness initiatives. Culture Amp[57] is one such company that is leading the way in innovative ways to assist companies to better support their people and improve employee engagement and productivity. Rise[58] is a Canadian-based company that provides similar services and also produces useful reports on wellness programs, diversity and inclusion strategies and employee engagement. In 2016, recruitment firm Robert Walters[59] conducted a study which found that sixty-four percent of job applicants said they would be more likely to apply for a position if the company promoted its health and wellness program in the job advertisement, and we know that Millennials are far more conscious about things such as an organization's corporate social responsibility, diversity and inclusion strategies and employee benefits and workplace policies, including those around wellness.

---

57. http://www.cultureamp.com/

58. https://risepeople.com/

59. https://www.robertwalters.us/

Millennials are also increasingly seeking occupations that provide work-life balance and are prioritizing work with a purpose. Analytics companies such as Qualtrix[60] and Gallup[61] are also able to provide similar data to companies around salaries, benefits and their link to engagement, loyalty, satisfaction, and productivity. Many of these organizations have workplace psychologists on staff that are ready to assist clients to navigate these complex issues and eliminate some of the guesswork, as their database generally includes a sampling of information covering a substantial number of employers globally.

The cost to business of not prioritizing employee wellness are substantial. In 2017, Gallup released the results of their fourth annual survey that revealed that only thirteen percent of employees globally feel engaged at work[62], and the biggest roadblock that employees face in feeling healthier and happier is the workplace culture, which encompasses direction from the top and the organization's people management and employee wellness strategies. In 2016, the Global Wellness Institute[63] released a report titled *The Future of Wellness at Work[64]*.

As outlined in the report, their research found that "only 9 percent of the global workforce has access to some form of wellness program at work. The breakdown in penetration: North America 52 percent of employees, Europe 23 percent, Middle East/North Africa 7 percent, Latin America/Caribbean 5 percent, Asia 5 percent, and Sub-Saharan Africa 1 percent. The U.S., where companies pay for employee healthcare, is by far the largest market and the greatest innovator, but as chronic disease skyrockets globally, and healthcare costs (paid via taxes) spike in markets like Europe, the Global Wellness Institute predicts significant growth in global workplace wellness spending in the next decade".

We are now in 2021 and as we all know, as a result of the COVID-19 global pandemic, in additional to physical illness, one of the side-effects has been a significant impact on mental health.

---

60. http://www.qualtrics.com/

61. https://www.gallup.com/

62. https://community.virginpulse.com/state-of-the-industry-employee-engagement-2018

63. https://globalwellnessinstitute.org

64. https://globalwellnessinstitute.org/industry-research/the-future-of-wellness-at-work/

The situation today is far worse than it was in 2016 when the Global Wellness Institute prepared the report, but its message remains the same – employee unwellness at work represents a significant cost to business. As of 2019, the cost of unwellness at work was estimated at $2.2 trillion annually or twelve percent of Gross Domestic Product and work-related stress alone can cost up to $300 billion a year[65].

As outlined in **Your Stories**, providing employees with flexibility or leave when needed to assist with grief, healing, or symptoms such as pain and discomfort associated with endometriosis, ovarian cysts, fibroids, or menopause, does not have to mean that there is a decline in productivity. In fact, in many cases, providing time to heal will result in the exact opposite – more productive employees when they return to work healed and refreshed. This is the whole premise behind mental health days. Taking a day when needed, to rest and replenish our internal supply of energy, is something that is needed by everybody. Just as we cannot expect to run a car on one tank of gas forever, the same rule applies to our bodies and minds. There is only so long the vehicle can continue without rest before damage will occur.

It surprises me that so many companies are fearful when someone asks for flexibility at work. Workplace flexibility is something I have seen vary significantly from one country to the next and even from one industry to another. Because much of my professional working life has been split between time in Australia and the U.S., one of the things that I have discovered is that employers in Australia tend to have a fundamental distrust of work-from-home arrangements (although COVID-19 has forced this issue in recent days), and employees generally need to earn trust first.

In contrast, in the U.S., employers are often more willing to provide flexibility in the first place, but will remove it if, or when, trust is broken. Work productivity can be measured and so I am often perplexed as to why such a negative connotation is applied to requests for flexibility. I often think back to one of the law firms that I worked for in Australia. I remember the head partner of the

---

65. https://allwork.space/2019/03/these-statistics-prove-that-wellness-improves-the-workplace-experience

team who positioned his office in a location where he had a clear view to watch when each person would enter or leave each day. If you arrived later than 8.30am or left before 6pm, he would glare at you and refuse to speak to you for days. That partner was the very definition of unapproachable and a very poor leader. Needless to say, I was miserable in that job and in a more flexible and supportive environment I quickly thrived.

For all of the reasons outlined, the cost of employee benefits and wellness initiatives is also something that is often miscalculated and for those companies that are merely trying to be profitable, these things are often just viewed as a cost that detracts from profit. However, that view is misguided because, as the numerous studies and research shows, there are other significant benefits to the organization through reduced costs and increased productivity which ultimately lead to improved profits in many cases.

In a 2017 study that was conducted by the University of California, Los Angeles (UCLA), Anderson School of Management, of those who were surveyed, it was found that sick employees and healthy individuals who improved their health increased productivity by about ten percent as a result of employee wellness program participation and post-program health changes[66]. The study does note that the sample included a small number of respondents, but nonetheless demonstrates the link between wellness, motivation, and ability.

I once heard a founder of a company make a comment about the air conditioning being too high in a workplace and she said she would always turn it down or off when she was there to save costs. I remember feeling horrified at the time that I heard it, but also fascinated by the comment because, as a woman, I would have expected she would be more understanding of her employees who might have really relied on that cool air.

For example, women who are pregnant or going through menopause often experience higher body temperatures or hot flushes. I have thought about that comment a lot, as it is an example

66. https://papers.ssrn.com/sol3/papers.cfm?abstract_id=2811785

of such a small situation that probably seems so insignificant to that founder, yet I could imagine exactly how I would feel if I was in that workplace, and I was sitting there when that happened. Would I resign from my employment as a result of something like that? No, probably not. Would I be unhappy, irritated, annoyed, or even angry or resentful of my employer? Yes, I absolutely would feel all of those things and those types of emotions and thoughts take energy – energy that is diverted away from being productive at your job.

I may also need to get up and go to the bathroom more frequently to cool down or change my clothes or go to the kitchen more often for cool water. Now, stop and think about just how many small and seemingly insignificant decisions are made in workplaces around the world like this every single day and imagine just how significant the impact is of these decisions on employee productivity. Makes you think, doesn't it?

IF WOMEN ALREADY HAVE A HARDER TIME AT WORK, WHY WOULD WE WANT TO HIGHLIGHT OUR DIFFERENCES?

This is a hard one because on some level, the women who ask me this are right. We are in a difficult situation right now because there are so many challenges that women face every single day and the workplace playing field is definitely not an even surface. It is tilted heavily with men at one end and women at the other. However, change cannot happen by being silent. There is power in speaking out publicly and in binding groups together on common issues.

Speaking out about our differences does not have to simply be in the context of a specific personal issue. In fact, much like the way in which preventative health works, this is how we should be approaching this issue. A good place to start is with miscarriage, because we know that there are high numbers of women who will be affected by miscarriage at some point in their life. We should also not forget about the effects on men either – miscarriage impacts the mental health of men as well. When you add these two things together, the figures are overwhelming and strongly indicate why all employers should be doing something to assist their employees when they are impacted by a miscarriage.

The reality is that employees are human and their experiences at work are therefore inevitably going to be impacted by the things that are happening in their personal lives – good and bad. Women are representative of almost half of the workforce, yet the reality of our experiences are largely being ignored. If we want to move forward towards equality, then we cannot continue to remain silent about our differences. It is those differences that need to be celebrated, supported and encouraged to strengthen our ability to succeed.

Differences in opinion and ideas are what lead to innovation, and they are the cornerstone of why diverse teams outperform those that are less diverse. There is unfortunately a stigma attached to 'difference', which we need to get better at overcoming, and the only way to do this is by talking more openly about these issues. Yes, men and women are different. That is the reality that we have been told many times before through self-help books such as Men Are from Mars, Women Are from Venus[67], a book that took on almost cult-like status after its release in 1992, and He's Just Not That Into You[68] which was also later made into a movie. We seem quite willing to accept that we are different when it comes to personal relationships, but in the workplace, our differences are all but forgotten and certainly not openly accepted and acknowledged without a negative connotation being attached.

So, why is it that we seem so stuck on moving past this outdated view? Well, a lot of it comes back to our ingrained bias and the views and ideas that we have been conditioned to believe as a result of the struggles of so many women before us in workplaces all over the world. As girls have had to fight their way into schools and universities throughout history and women have been subjected to adversity when entering male-dominated professions, those women have learnt to fight to survive. Much of their efforts were historically

67. https://en.wikipedia.org/wiki/Men_Are_from_Mars,_Women_Are_from_Venus
68. https://en.wikipedia.org/wiki/He%27s_Just_Not_That_Into_You

focused on proving that their capabilities were equal to those of their male colleagues.

These women are to be admired and respected because they paved the way for us all, but like everything, time has moved forward, and we are now at a point where we need to demand more. We have established ourselves within the workforce and have demonstrated that we belong there, but we are now in an era where we want to see true equality. In my view, that can only be achieved by recognizing our differences and demanding that they be better supported and, indeed, celebrated.

When three brilliant African American women at NASA in 1961 – Katherine Johnson, Dorothy Vaughan and Mary Jackson – became the brains behind the launch of astronaut John Glenn into orbit, they were faced with much adversity, merely because they were women, and women of color at that. However, did that stop them despite their differences and in the knowledge that what they were trying to do would be hard? No. It did not and today we admire those women and everything that they achieved for space travel, women, and people of color.

At that time though, their actions were extreme. They were in contrast to the norm and what people at that time believed and felt comfortable with but, as we know, they led us to something much greater – the start of more opportunities and respect for women and people of color within NASA. The same applies here. We need women to stop fearing their differences and their workplaces and find ways to explain our differences and demonstrate how workplaces can better support women to succeed by enhancing our strengths.

Contrary to popular belief, the most important differences between men and women in the workplace are not related to women prioritizing family responsibilities, lacking confidence, or negotiating poorly. Rather, the most significant differences lie in the way in which men and women are treated and the lack of appreciation of the roles and responsibilities of men and women – as well as the unique health issues that women face. The differences between men and women are not related to attitudes, behaviors, or capabilities – and this is absolutely critical to understand, because it is the source of much of the fear and negative connotations around 'differences'. These beliefs are **what hold women back every single day** and we all must destroy these myths, because the science actually shows us that women and men are far more similar than they are different in terms of attitudes, capabilities and skills.

This is why having discussions within organizations about these issues is so important. To address this issue, an organization should be looking at its practices, systems, and policies to analyze how they are creating different experiences for their male and female employees at work. Ultimately, what we need to get to is a situation where an organization's practices, systems and policies better support their men and women to succeed because they recognize the differences in experiences, not their characteristics or abilities.

I VALUE MY PRIVACY ABOUT MY PERSONAL HEALTH ISSUES

Some people are really private. I get it. I am clearly not one of those people or I wouldn't be sharing my story with you so publicly in this book. However, like everyone, I too have certain things about myself that are private, and that I don't want to share. That is completely reasonable, but whenever I think about an issue and whether I will share it, I try to stop and think about the benefits of doing so. Firstly, sharing our story allows us to get our feelings out into the open. It provides us with a way to share with others and get feedback and support. It also helps us to find communities of others with similar experiences and as humans we crave this type of connection. When we find a community that we can relate to, we learn, grow, and often heal as well.

Secondly, rarely is it possible to get help or support without offering someone a glimpse of what you are going through. Employers are not mind readers. However, they do act on what they see. If you are struggling at work because of a health issue but you don't tell anyone and your performance drops, don't expect your employer to continue just letting it slide. It is far better to speak up and explain what you are going through because when you do that, employers are generally a lot more willing to give you some leniency for a period of time.

Until you speak up, you also have no idea what your employer might say or do to try to support you. And, as I have mentioned, offering up some of your own suggestions can really assist to shape the conversation as well. Because employers are not medical experts and most managers will not have experienced whatever issue you are personally going through, they may not know what support is going to best assist you. Therefore, explaining the issue and offering some solutions with explanations of why it will help you to continue to perform is the best way to approach your employer for help.

In my view, the most important reason to speak up about your health issues, is because of the way it can open dialogs about these issues and ultimately help other women – if you can influence change within your organization. That was the main driving force for me. Because I know how difficult it can be for any woman going through fertility struggles, child-loss, endometriosis and menopause, I want to share my story to explain to employers just how significant an impact they can have on a person's health journey, and why the support they provide or withhold will directly influence an employee's ability to succeed at work.

I want to show companies that there are far better ways to help women in the workplace and I hope to do that by sharing my story, explaining the data that is out there to support my theories and then providing some practical tips to get started on implementing better support for women within every organization.

I appreciate that not every woman feels that they are in a position to speak up, if and when they are struggling at work. That is why I also believe women leaders have a particularly important role to play here. We have a responsibility to speak up about these issues within our organizations and not just when issues arise, but also more proactively. Change often happens as a result of crisis, and because people have a general fear of change and the unknown, when that does happen, it often occurs quickly as a means to resolve an immediate issue. Well, I would like to challenge you all now to take action promptly because, in my view, we are in a situation of crisis.

We are rapidly going backwards on workplace gender equality. In 2021, the gender pay gap widened and as a result of the COVID-19 global pandemic, we have seen women withdraw from the workforce at higher rates than ever before in history. This means that there will be less women in workplaces that are able to improve diversity on boards and in the C-Suite (executive-level managers). This is a situation of crisis and one that we simply must recognize now, before the situation worsens, and take active steps to address – but it is going to require more women speaking up about this issue, and supporting other women to start effecting real change. What is more important? The future of all women, or your own privacy? I know what I think.

HEALTH ISSUES ARE NOT A WORKPLACE ISSUE, OR ARE THEY?

Every day, humans across the globe spend anywhere from one-third to one-half of their waking hours at work. Our workforce is aging too, which is also impacting employee wellness because, as people age, health issues tend to increase. It is estimated that 18 percent of the labor force globally will be over fifty-five by 2030[69].

Various research studies have estimated the costs of work-related stress around the world: $650 billion in Europe, $3.9 billion in Australia, $2.8 billion in Canada, and $300 billion in the United States[70]. Studies have also found that disengaged employees are less productive, more likely to steal from their company, negatively influence their coworkers, miss more workdays, and drive customers away. Healthy, well-rested and motivated employees on the other hand, make better decisions and are more effective and productive.

69. ILO; WHO; Gallup; Gallup-Healthways; Towers-Watson; Tampere University of Technology/Workplace Safety & Health Institute Singapore/VTT Technical Research Centre of Finland

70. Hassard, J., et al (2014). Calculating the cost of work-related stress and psychosocial risks – A Literature Review. Bilbao, Spain: European Agency for Safety and Health at Work. https://osha.europa.eu/en/tools-and-publications/publications/literature_reviews/calculating-the-cost-of-work-relatedstress-and-psychosocial-risks.

Importantly though, work also has the ability to impact the symptoms associated with health conditions, for example, through stress – or improve health, such as depression and anxiety, by providing people with purpose and something to commit to each day.

Rapidly rising rates of chronic disease are escalating healthcare costs around the world. The World Economic Forum and Harvard School of Public Health in their report, *The Global Economic Burden of Non-Communicable Diseases*[71], estimated in September 2011 that major chronic diseases and mental illness would result in a projected cumulative $47 trillion in lost economic output globally from 2011–2030. This figure is likely much higher now as a result of the COVID-19 global pandemic, and importantly, it does not factor in the costs associated with lost productivity or absenteeism.

These and the many other examples of the statistics related to employee health and wellness, including the number of women who suffer – often silently – from various illnesses, diseases, and health conditions, clearly show that women's health issues are a workplace issue. It is unreasonable and unrealistic to think that an employee can simply 'switch-off' whatever symptoms they are experiencing once they enter the workplace, or sit in front of their computer and switch into work mode. The lines between work and home are also being increasingly blurred. More people than ever before have been forced to convert their homes into their office space as a result of the global pandemic. With 24/7 connectivity, there are more instances of employee burnout which leads to reduced productivity, and this increases turnover. The employers that recognize this and start finding better ways to support their employees, now and into the future, are the ones that will attract the best talent, retain their staff for longer, perform better than their competitors and place their businesses in a stronger position to achieve longevity.

There is ample data that shows us that companies that infuse wellness into their corporate cultures experience improved performance. The Great Place to Work® Institute, which recognizes

---

71.http://www3.weforum.org/docs/WEF_Harvard_HE_GlobalEconomicBurdenNonCommunicableDiseases_2011

the 100 top companies in the United States for workplace culture, found that 'great workplaces' had sixty-five percent lower employee turnover, and stock market returns that were two times higher than industry peers from 1997-2014[72].

Companies appearing on Glassdoor.com[73] 'best places to work' list (based on ratings derived directly from employee feedback) outperformed the S&P 500 by 115.6 percent from 2009-2015; conversely, companies with the lowest employee ratings on Glassdoor.com significantly underperformed the market[74]. Yet so many companies continue to prioritize short-term gains. This is a short-sighted approach and one that I believe will be unsustainable in the future. Job applicants, employees and customers are demanding more of companies and actively seeking out those that are more socially conscious about the environment and people. Customers are becoming more interested in the story and meaning behind a brand and consumers are increasingly making conscious choices to boycott companies that exploit employees and the environment.

We all have a role to play here – employees included. If you approach your employer with problems without offering any solutions, then you may be seen as the problem and that is a mindset that we definitely want to avoid. I myself was guilty of this for a long time but eventually, once I changed the narrative, I had different conversations which generated far better outcomes for both parties.

We need to start being open about the health issues we are experiencing and how the symptoms are impacting us at work, because this is the only way to educate others. We cannot refuse to involve men in the conversation because we are concerned about disclosing our personal health issue, yet expect them to simply understand what we are going through. Men don't experience menstruation or pregnancy or menopause and so how can we expect them to know

72. Great Place to Work® Institute (n.d.). What are the benefits? The ROI on workplace culture. http://www.greatplacetowork.com/our-approach/whatare-the-benefits-great-workplaces. See also: Edmans, A. (2011). Does the stock market fully value intangibles? Employee satisfaction and equity prices. Journal of Financial Economics, 101, 621-640. http://faculty.london.edu/aedmans/Rowe.pdf.

73. https://www.glassdoor.com/

74. Chamberlain, A. (2015, March). Does Company Culture Pay Off? Analyzing Stock Performance of "Best Places to Work" Companies. Mill Valley, CA: Glassdoor.com. https://research-content.glassdoor.com/app/uploads/sites/2/2015/05/GD_Report_1.pdf.

what these things are like and how they can impact us at work if we don't start talking about these things and explain?

It is absolutely critical to involve men in the wider discussions within organizations around female health issues and the workplace as well. Equality cannot be achieved without including men in the conversation, and also getting them on board and invested. Employers need to provide people with a safe environment and the tools and resources needed to be able to have those conversations and foster cultures that break down and eliminate the stigma attached to women's health issues. Employers also need to start researching and looking at the data and really trying to understand it, and then take steps to educate their boards, executive and management teams. We need to infuse every level of management with knowledge about the measurable, tangible cost benefits to leading with, and creating a culture that fosters employee health and wellness – one that caters more specifically for each employee and their individual experiences and needs in the workplace.

The Importance of Mentors and Sponsors

Female mentorship and sponsorship by both men and women in the workplace is more important than ever before. As the number of women in the workforce is declining and we are going backwards in the progress we had achieved towards closing the gender equality gap – mentorship and sponsorship must play a key role in promoting the retention and upward mobility of women in the workplace.

Studies by Catalyst[75] and Harvard Business Review[76] have shown that women who have sponsors are more likely to advance in their careers. A recent study by PayScale found that women who have a sponsor are paid ten percent more than women without one[77]. It is more important for women to have strong and supportive mentors and sponsors so they can see what is possible by watching and learning from the steps that have been taken by other successful women.

Sponsors also play a crucial role because without a voice at the table where the decisions are being made, in many workplace environments it can be extremely difficult for a woman to get noticed and considered for opportunities and promotions. Equally, if we want to move closer towards closing the gender equality gap, then we simply cannot hope to do so without men taking on mentor and sponsor roles as well, in addition to more broadly leading by example.

So, what is the difference between a mentor and a sponsor? Well, a mentor can be anyone in a position of experience. A mentor passes on their knowledge, provides advice and support, and guides an employee along their career journey. A sponsor on the other hand is someone within your organization who is in a position of power

---

75. https://www.catalyst.org/

76. https://hbr.org/

77. https://www.shrm.org/hr-today/news/hr-magazine/winter2019/pages/why-male-leaders-should-mentor-women.aspx

and is able to advocate for you when decisions are being made. A sponsor is vested in assisting you to progress upward and they will assist in your professional development.

Not everyone will have a mentor in their lifetime and not everyone will have a sponsor. Sometimes sponsors might also play a silent role and a person may not even realize that they have a sponsor at the table, advocating on their behalf. Sponsorship therefore does not have to be a formal arrangement and it is something that every leader can do for another employee who shows potential. Mentorship, on the other hand, generally cannot occur without both parties participating knowingly in the process. Whether a mentor or a sponsor is right for you will depend on the circumstances. I have never had sponsor, or at least one that I have known about, so my view is that a sponsor is certainly not crucial to succeed. However, sponsors can be invaluable assets and if you are presented with such an opportunity, jump!

Mentors also serve a crucial role in the professional and personal development of another person by enabling a person to share ideas, brainstorm, practice and sometimes even to vent frustrations in a safe environment where they can be redirected into ultimately more constructive conversations. I have had a number of mentors during my career. Unfortunately, only one of them was a woman, as my experience has been that it is more difficult to find a female mentor – which is always something that has floored me.

Women leaders simply must step up and do better in this area. Not only is it crucial that we lead by setting good examples for other women to follow, but it is equally important we take the time to seek out other young women and men to mentor. Mentoring women assists them by providing the skills and tools to navigate the culture of the organization, and mentoring young men helps to shape the culture, as those new hires will one day end up being the seasoned, experienced employees that are making decisions within organizations.

Because it has been so difficult for many women to climb to the top of the career ladder, there is research that shows that women leaders can actually be tougher on other women within their organizations. In a study conducted by Skyline International[78], more than 1,000 professionals were surveyed on leadership qualities, and in doing so it was found that women rated the effectiveness of other women lower, fifty-seeven percent of the time regarding workplace competencies, compared to men at fourteen percent.

An article in Forbes in 2016, *Women In The Workplace: Are Women Tougher On Other Women?*[79] says: "According to a 2007 survey from the Employment Law Alliance, of the 45 percent of people who said they had been bullied in the workplace, 40 percent said they were bullied by women. That, in and of itself, does not prove women are more likely to torment other women. But a 2014 report from the Workplace Bullying Institute claims that women who were considered workplace bullies targeted other women 68 percent of the time. Sindell also uncovered a 2011 report from the American Management Association which declared that about 95 percent of women have been 'tormented' by another woman during their careers. Says Sindell: 'Whereas men who are bullies are equal-opportunity tormentors, they weren't directed at any particular segment. Our study really reinforces some of those findings.'"

As the article discusses, one of the reasons for this is competition. Younger employees who present promise can represent a threat to more seasoned employees, especially as younger, newly educated employees often enter the workplace with fresh, innovative ideas and tend to have much better knowledge and skills in the area of new technologies. The other reason why women can develop a hardened approach to the management of other women is that some women who have made it to the top, having faced challenges and opposition along the way, end up developing a mindset of, "Well, I had to work extra hard to get there so you can too". Ultimately, this is a cycle that we simply must break if we are ever to achieve gender equality and we need women leaders and future leaders to remember this and pave the way for an easier journey for the generations that follow behind us.

---

78. https://skylineg.com/

79. https://www.forbes.com/sites/karstenstrauss/2016/07/18/women-in-the-workplace-are-women-tougher-on-other-women/?sh=5c7e068547ea

Closing the gender gap is not about providing an easier ride for women when compared to the men within an organization. It is about ensuring that future generations of women will have the same opportunities as men to succeed at work, through taking account of the significant differences that exist between the roles of women, the challenges faced by women and accordingly, the needs of women in order to place them in the best possible position to succeed at work.

It is about ensuring that an employee will be selected or promoted based on results, skills, and experience – that gender will play no part in the decision – and that men and women will receive equal pay for equal work. It is also about ensuring that women are no longer subjected to the type of sexual harassment so many women have suffered in the workplace, from leering, sexual comments and threats – to even worse, situations of abuse – this type of conduct has never, ever been okay and we simply must demand tougher enforcement and penalties for those who engage in any of these types of behavior in the future. Mentoring future generations plays a key role in the elimination of sexual harassment in the workplace.

I strongly believe that many of my successes would not have been possible without the support and guidance of my mentors throughout the years. One in particular, Mike, has been there with me every step of my career, right back to my first year of practice as a lawyer. He has been there for me to listen to me and guide me whenever I have needed his help or support. He has commiserated with me in times of hardship and has celebrated my successes as if they were his own. It is because of Mike, and the other mentors that have assisted me along the way, that I understand how important it is to similarly give back to future generations by sharing my story, my knowledge, and the lessons that I have learnt along the way. Mentoring takes work for sure, but just as my own mentors took the time to invest in me, I believe that I too have an obligation to make the time for future generations.

There is another unexpected benefit to mentoring and that is that often the mentor will end up learning things from the mentee as well. I know that this has certainly been true in my own experience, and I am fairly sure that my mentor Mike would say the same thing about me. Mentoring another person also helps to develop your leadership skills and this is something I think every single manager should strive to continuously improve.

Workplace culture changes over time and differs from one organization to another. New generations of employees enter organizations and communication and management styles need to continually adapt over time to accommodate the differences that exist from one generation to the next. Laws continually change and with them, expectations of employees and employers. For all of these reasons and more, leadership skills should be fluid and continually developed, to account for each unique situation as the workplace structure and culture changes.

Mentoring also provides you with new perspectives on issues. I always think back to my boss Karl, at Hall & Wilcox, when I think about this. Karl remains a good friend of mine to this day and I credit him for teaching me business development skills as a young lawyer. When I think back to some of the meetings I used to have with Karl, he would guide and instruct me on various issues, and every so often, I would come back to him with a fresh idea or a new perspective. We would often debate about whatever my idea was and sometimes he would stop, I would see him think and then he would say something like, "Okay. Let's try it. I haven't thought about it that way. Maybe that is better."

Karl is an example of a great manager and a good mentor, because he was not always fixed on his ideas. He was willing to provide me with an opportunity to try new ways of doing things. Sometimes a new idea will succeed and sometimes it won't, but a good manager should be willing to let an employee try, and succeed or learn from the mistakes. That is the type of leadership example we should all be demonstrating because ultimately, it is the leadership style we need future generations to carry forward as well.

Mentoring can also be a really rewarding experience. The personal satisfaction you feel watching another person succeed is extremely gratifying. It also provides an opportunity for self-reflection. It enables you to sit back and consider all you have achieved and the journey to get there. This type of knowledge is invaluable to a mentee, but it is also a very useful exercise for a manager to do personally. Sometimes we get so caught up in the stresses of life and we can also get weighed down with the burden of whatever is on our plates that we forget to stop and think about our own achievements. I know I am personally guilty of this at times.

There are some days when I feel the weight of the world on my shoulders as I try to manage my busy workload, my board position responsibilities and be there for my children as much as I possibly can be (oh and also write a book!). On those days I can easily find myself slipping into a mindset of, *how can I possibly get all of this done*?! I start to feel the onset of panic mode and then I quickly stop myself. *Have I ever fallen apart before? Have I ever not gotten through it all eventually? Are my children going to die or end up sick or injured if I am not able to be there for that 1 class, when I have not missed one for many weeks? Are they going to think I am a terrible mother if I can't read them a story tonight?* I go through all of these questions in my head, and when the answer to each one is inevitably *No!*, I immediately calm down.

The next thing I do is create a list and tick off each item as I complete them. This helps immensely. I cannot recommend this enough. I love lists. I use old-school notebooks, the Notes page on my iPhone, as well as a whiteboard. If it wasn't for all of my lists, I would be lost. It keeps me organized and makes my life feel manageable even on those chaotic days. Putting the list into days also helps to break down what I think is going to be achievable on each particular day – but I also have to be flexible in my approach because, as a lawyer, client emergencies can arise at any time. Life happens sometimes, so don't get too rigid in the approach. Do what you can when you can and try to keep on track. Use time wisely.

I have seen many people who complain that they are time poor, yet spend hours complaining about not having enough time, or about their co-worker or boss who is making their life difficult. I have been guilty of this in the past, but not anymore. When I have spare time, I use it well. Time is extremely valuable. We only get a certain amount of it, and I plan to make the most of it all, as productively as possible.

These are the types of skills that are extremely valuable to a mentee. Mentoring does not have to be just about teaching skills within your particular industry. It is just as much about teaching life skills, communication skills and management skills, and with years of experience in the workplace, we all end up with many of these skills to teach others.

THE ROLE OF MEN

Men are critical to the success of any diversity and inclusion strategy, and they are crucial to finding the solution to the workplace gender gap. Put simply, men must be part of the solution. They need to be our allies in our fight to close the gender equality gap. I believe that men are also the most underutilized resource that we have within organizations – and while most of us look to successful women to assist with this journey, as there are significantly more men in leadership roles and positions of power. We need to find ways to connect with and recruit more men to be champions for the cause. Seeking out male mentors is a great way to do that.

As the 2019 Women in the Workplace study by McKinsey & Co. and LeanIn.org[80] suggests, one way to ensure that all employees are receiving an equal distribution of a manager's time, support and guidance is to implement key performance indicators or measurable outcomes that track this. Organizations can also go a step further and specifically impose mentorship and sponsorship obligations on their managers and executive teams. As David Smith, the co-author of *Athena Rising: How and Why Men Should Mentor Women* (Bibliomotion, 2016) says, one of the benefits of men mentoring women is that they often find that their contacts expand as they end up with networks that they would not otherwise have access to. For a man in sales, in a leadership role or who is responsible for recruitment, this can be an invaluable benefit of being in a mentor or sponsor relationship.

In addition to the importance of men in leadership roles mentoring women, equally important is the mentoring and coaching

---

80. https://www.mckinsey.com/featured-insights/diversity-and-inclusion/women-in-the-workplace#

of younger generations of men. This is a critical component of improving conditions and opportunities for women in the workplace for the next generation and beyond. It is also key to breaking down the gender biases that we know currently exist today in the workplace. There needs to be more concerted efforts to set up and structure mentoring efforts for men and women. We tend to teach our young employees about the skills needed to do the job, as well as how to effectively work with and manage colleagues from all backgrounds.

BUILDING A MENTORSHIP PROGRAM WITHIN YOUR ORGANIZATION

There are many benefits of developing a formal, structured mentoring program with an organization. A mentor program can create happier, more loyal employees who feel better informed and valued. It can also produce more effective leaders. As a good leader will be able to get the best out of their people, this is ultimately good news for an organization's production and profitability. Companies can only ever benefit from a skilled workforce, and when communication occurs broadly across functions and teams, this generally creates improved teamwork and results because employees have a greater understanding of the inner workings of the organization and how each component fits together. It also helps to reduce cross-over or double-up on work and roles, which inevitably occurs in every organization to some extent, and it provides an opportunity to transfer knowledge organically. This essentially becomes an insurance plan if someone leaves suddenly, and is a useful tool that could form the basis of any organization's succession plan.

So, now that you have the business case or the 'why', what should a mentoring program look like? Well, it is going to be different for every organization and industry. However, there are some key tips that I can share:

- **It should be voluntary for employees:** With the exception of managers and executives, who in my view, should be required to mentor or support more junior employees.

Apart from this requirement, this type of mentorship program should otherwise be voluntary. Not every employee wants to be mentored. Not every employee has a desire to progress through the organization or become a manager, and an employee's own desires for their career should be respected. If an employee does not enjoy the responsibilities associated with a leadership or management role then it is probably not the right career path for them. Employers and managers should listen to their employees when they either say this through their words or actions. Forcing an employee to go down a career path that they are not interested in inevitably ends in disaster. These people become resentful, are unmotivated, and they are often terrible managers because they never wanted to be there to begin with – it was just a progression that they were pushed into.

- **It should be open to all employees, at any level:** Many organizations reserve training courses and other benefits such as mentoring programs and business development coaching for their higher-level employees. This is something that I have seen consistently in many law firms, and in my view, it is a mistake. Just as we teach skills to children from infancy so that they become familiar and second nature as the child grows and develops, we should adopt the same approach to new employees entering the workplace. Yes, the mentoring may look a little different at each stage in a person's career, but the importance is just the same no matter the level, because ultimately, the aim is to assist employees to progress right from the early stages of their career through to wherever they ultimately end up at the end of their working life. Rather than trying to teach employees skills once they reach a certain point in their career, I think that we should be teaching them certain skills from day one so that it becomes second nature. Ingraining mentorship from an early stage in a person's career will also assist to create a cycle of mentees that will eventually become mentors and this, in turn, starts to change culture on a wider scale.

- **Match mentors and mentees from different teams, departments, or functions within the business:** Mentors will often seek out mentees with whom they share similar traits. It is human nature to be attracted to others who resemble us. Mentoring presents opportunities for people to move outside of their comfort zone and learn different perspectives from others with different backgrounds, experiences, etc. It provides an opportunity to see new perspectives. It also enables more communication and collaboration across a wider section of the organization as mentors and mentees will gain a greater understanding of the various functions and roles within the organization and how they each work together to create the final product or service that is ultimately delivered to the end-user or client. This type of knowledge can significantly increase productivity and it is something that I have personally experienced first-hand. Within my current firm, Littler, we do a fantastic job of mentoring our younger lawyers and teaching them about the various functions and capabilities within the firm by including them in firm events, trainings, workshops, and conferences. In many other firms, lawyers will only be included in events, conferences, and any client-facing meetings once they reach a certain stage in their career. In my view, this is the wrong approach as it limits their exposure and professional growth. A partner in a law firm and a manager or executive in an organization are certainly not the only people who can bring in a client or close a deal. When I was just a second-year lawyer, I had already started gaining clients of my own – and I am not unique. We need to encourage our new employees in these areas from day one, because ultimately, an employee's success at any level, equals success for the organization as well. Involving employees at all stages of their career and from any team or function also creates far better knowledge within teams. This way, if an employee in the sales team is asked a question about the organization's technology for example, the employee may know exactly who to ask to get an answer, without having to spend valuable time investigating.

- **Match based on skills gaps:** Another way to create effective mentor relationships is to conduct an analysis of the areas of strengths and weaknesses of both your managers and potential mentees. Rather than randomly assigning mentors and mentees, or allowing these relationships to develop organically, with a formal mentor program, it can benefit both parties to do some analysis first to determine (a) the areas of strength of both parties; and (b) the gaps in skills and experience which represent the areas where a mentoring relationship would be of benefit. After conducting this type of analysis and matching parties accordingly, it will enable the mentor and mentee to exchange valuable skills and insights with one another and may also end up mutually beneficial in different ways to each party.

- **Support and value the program:** There is little point putting any policy or program in place within an organization if it is ultimately not given the support and value that it needs to succeed. If a manager doesn't see that an organization values a mentoring program, the manager may end up cancelling meetings with their mentee as things come up and their workload gets busy. For a mentor relationship to be worthwhile and valuable to both parties, it requires commitment on both sides, and accountability assists to ensure that the parties maintain this commitment for the duration of the relationship. Creating the space, time and support for mentors and mentees to commit to the process is crucial for any formal mentor program to succeed. Introducing mentorship key performance indicators for your managers is a great way to do this. Supporting mentor relationships also makes business sense for another reason: it assists with the development of an organization's succession planning. Having executive team members and managers mentor lower-level managers who are coming up through the ranks, provides a valuable transfer of knowledge within an organization and potentially, future opportunities for those individuals to step into the roles of executives and managers as they leave the organization for other opportunities or retire.

- **Provide training for mentors and mentees:** Not everyone knows how to be a great mentor or mentee from day one, and each mentor relationship will be different, but for a person to get the most out of the relationship they need to understand how mentorships work, what the respective obligations and the role of each party are. Training can also assist the parties to understand what they can do if a mentor relationship isn't working. This might include terminating the relationship, talking through the issues, re-setting expectations or re-assigning the parties to a different mentor/mentee. Not every mentor relationship is going to be a perfect fit, and that's okay. Sometimes it is better for both parties to call it quits so that each respective party can find a more beneficial relationship. A mentorship also doesn't have to be long-term or last forever. In fact, it is rarely the case, and that is fine too. Mentorships may come to a natural conclusion as a person develops skills and experience, and their needs for support at work change. It is always best for a party to be honest and clear about this if they feel that the time has come to end the relationship for whatever reason.

MENTORING AT A BOARD LEVEL

One of the things we are in the process of implementing at a board level within one of the organizations I am a part of, is a mentoring program through a board sub-committee or advisory board. The idea behind this sprang from discussions we were having internally about how we could better support our female and minority employees, and further attract a more diverse workforce. As a result of those discussions, we each realized that in our own ways, we were already mentoring and sponsoring young people who showed potential, but for whatever reason weren't receiving opportunities we felt they would thrive in.

We decided we wanted to do more, and start putting some structure around this for the benefit of the organization and its future growth. We also understood that directors of a company have a limited lifespan. There will come a time when each of us will leave the board, and transferring our skills, knowledge and experience to other potential future board members would be a valuable tool that would place us ahead of most companies, simply because few organizations are doing anything like this.

As a result, we decided to establish board sub-committees or advisory boards which we will recruit by focusing on filling the positions with diverse members from all over the world. Why? Well, we genuinely want to learn about and listen to new perspectives, because we believe that this will make us a much better organization. To get the best out of our people we need to invest the time and resources to understand them. To learn about who they are, how they work and what they need at work and even beyond the workplace. We also want to learn from others outside of our industry. People who have different lived experiences than our own. We want to know what the challenges that people of color face in the workplace are, and some ways that we can assist to improve the workplace and our recruitment strategies to attract more employees of color.

We want to know the challenges that employees with disabilities face in the workplace and what tools would assist to improve the workplace experience for those employees. We want to know how we can better assist single parents or employees who are carers, and we want to hear the perspective of employees in the LGBTQ+ community and find ways to better attract, retain and support these employees as well. And, there is no better way to do this than to find, recruit and appoint people with all of these lived experiences to our advisory boards and sub-committees – so that we can start working on the solutions needed to move the needle towards workplace equality.

HOW TO FIND A MENTOR OR SPONSOR

The first step to finding a mentor is to work out some personal goals for yourself and your career, as this will help to shape your path and to determine what it is you are looking for in a mentor. This is also important as it will determine your expectations for the relationship. Both parties in a mentorship should be clear up front about what each person expects and wants out of the relationship, or it is unlikely to work.

The next step is to develop a list of the characteristics of your ideal mentor, some of the contacts in your network who you admire, and what skills, experience, or traits that you most admire, and why. Having a mentor within your own organization can be great but sometimes it is even better to be able to learn from people who are impartial and unbiased by the inner workings of it, and bounce your ideas and frustrations from others who have no relationships with the characters within it. A mentor who has experience in your particular field of expertise though can often assist. For those that are looking for mentoring and guidance in management and executive roles generally, the industry experience may not be as important.

Finding a mentor is a process. It is generally not something that happens overnight. It takes time to get to know someone and gain their attention and respect, so the first step is to reach out and start finding ways to have conversations with anyone you are targeting as a mentor, on topics that are of interest to them and within their area/s of expertise. Staying connected without annoying a person is key.

For example, continuing to check in and ask for advice on various topics every few months or a couple of times a year, attending events where you know the person is speaking and then sending an email to let them know how much you enjoyed their session are reasonable things to do that can open doors to further discussions. On the other hand, sending emails every week or so to ask random questions or directly asking someone who you don't know very well, "Will you be my mentor?" is unlikely to generate a positive response. Think about an appropriate way to start and continue communications with a potential mentor in order to build rapport first, before adopting a direct approach that may not end with a successful mentor match.

For mentors, I would encourage you to be open to approaches and start letting people know that you are open to mentoring. It is not easy to approach a person to mentor you, and having people publicly express that they are willing and available if the fit is right will remove some of the stress and anxiety that can be associated with finding a mentor. This is also another reason why formal mentor programs within organizations can really help.

Finding a sponsor can be a little more challenging than a mentor, because it requires someone to speak out publicly on your behalf, which ultimately has the potential to impact their own career if they do so and you disappoint. The first thing to note about finding a sponsor is that these are relationships built on mutual respect and trust, and therefore you will generally need to have some proven track record before a person will agree to be your sponsor.

You will need to show commitment, dedication, hard work, and some success and be seen as a person who is prepared to put yourself out there to find opportunities and be proactive in your approach. You need to make yourself valuable, and be willing to do not only what is asked of you or expected, but more. Ask questions constantly, inquire often and always strive to improve and grow. These are all qualities and attributes that will get you noticed and are the best ways to attract a sponsor who will want to work with you and support you on your journey. As you find your way to the top though, don't forget to look back for others that you too can similarly help along the way with their own journeys as well.

A mentor should always:

- Be prepared;
- Review any materials and online information prior to the call/ meeting;
- Be present during meetings (put away the cell phone!);
- Be on time;
- Acknowledge any conflicts up front;
- Do what you said you would do;
- Consider confidentiality issues (business, IP).

A mentee should always:

- Be prepared;
- Provide any briefing materials in advance, including the topics you want to cover (i.e., issues, challenges, goals, strategy etc.);
- Study mentor's background and experience prior to the call/meeting;
- Be on time;
- Be present during the call/meeting;
- Respect the mentor's time. Stick to the time allocated;
- Summarize next steps before the end of the call/meeting, if any;
- Get to know the mentor. Ask questions. Be interested. Be helpful if, and when, you can. Mentoring is a two-way street;
- Be respectful and considerate of boundaries. A mentor is a professional business contact. A mentor is generally not a friend to share your intimate secrets with.

What Innovative Companies Around the World Are Doing to Tackle this Issue

For any employee wellness policy, employee benefit or initiative to be effective, it should be implemented with the intention of improving employee's lives. Although there will certainly be flow-on benefits for the organization, these types of initiatives cannot be effectively implemented with business outcomes solely in mind. The primary purpose should not be to improve the company's reputation or merely tick a compliance box. Employee wellness initiatives will not be effective where they are intended to act as a veil to cover up demanding and unreasonable job expectations, or worse, as a means to gather private information about your employees.

In 2019, Yale University was sued as a result of its implementation of an employee wellness program that purported to be voluntary, but which penalized those who did not participate by deducting $25 a week from their salary[81]. Those employees who were opposed to the program argued that they did not want their personal information shared with the company and as failure to participate in the program would result in a financial penalty, it was not genuinely optional. Employees see right through an employer that is disingenuous. However, when implemented effectively, benefits, policies and programs that are well thought out and executed with the employees in mind can have significant value for the organization. And, as I have outlined in **Tackling the Opposition**, there are many benefits in doing so, including improved employee engagement, productivity, and profitability.

While it is great that more employers are talking about employee wellness at work, and mental health has become a common topic of discussion as a result of work-from-home mandates due to

---

81. https://www.shrm.org/ResourcesAndTools/hr-topics/benefits/Pages/workers-sue-Yale-University-over-workplace-wellness-penalties.aspx

COVID-19, declaring its importance is not enough to make people feel safe opening up about health issues or personal struggles. It doesn't educate employees about who they can go to if they need to discuss their issues or what they can do to ask for help, and what assistance is available to them. It also doesn't prepare managers for how to have conversations with their employee about these issues. The execution of the roll-out and ongoing management of any employee initiative is therefore just as important as the benefit itself.

Employees talk – often loudly and publicly through online platforms such as Glassdoor, where both current and former employees can go to rate companies either positively or negatively. Negative ratings on websites such as Yelp and Glassdoor have the potential to cause significant reputation and brand damage, and we frequently get clients contacting us in a panic, asking for us to help them to remove a poor rating. Unfortunately, it is virtually an impossible task, and once posted it is there for the world to see. This should not be the sole reason why a company seeks to implement a benefit that will market well to employees and job candidates, but it just serves as an additional reason why all organizations should prioritize the needs of its most important asset – its people.

Employee wellness is not a new phenomenon, but what I am suggesting is that we need to be thinking about it a bit differently and more broadly. Rather than merely offering yoga classes and providing healthy meals or fruit in the office (all of which are good things by the way!), I want employers to be thinking about benefits, flexible work arrangements and policies that are tailored more specifically to employees and their needs and experiences to better assist them to succeed.

Benefits and programs that think about physical and mental health, work-life balance, equal pay and benefits, the way in which we work, and employee motivations. The following companies are a mere sampling of some of the organizations that are doing just that. Some are employers, some are service providers and others are changemakers that are advocating for better opportunities for women.

WORK180

WORK180 was founded by Australian entrepreneurs, Valeria Ignatieva and Gemma Lloyd, to help women easily identify organizations committed to gender equity, diversity, and inclusion.

To be featured on the platform, employers must first show they meet WORK180's minimum standards related to important areas like parental leave, flexible work options and health care. If they do, they get the right to show the WORK180 badge across all their branding, a seal of approval that identifies them as an 'Endorsed Employer for ALL Women'. They also get to showcase their employer profile and vacancies on WORK180's transparent job board.

This is great for women seeking new opportunities as it offers visibility of open roles in companies who have been thoroughly vetted, and are committed to progress. It's just one example of how WORK180 is delivering on its mission *'to raise organizational standards so that all women can choose workplaces where they will thrive'*.

For employers, getting endorsed by WORK180 also gives them access to additional benefits to support their goals. WORK180's gender equity index helps companies to benchmark themselves against other organizations in their region, and identify what they should focus on next. WORK180 also runs regular campaigns to help raise awareness of employers who are leading the way with progressive policies, benefits and initiatives, often spotlighting the stories of women employees who have experienced this support firsthand. These are the kinds of things that can get missed when companies are busy focusing on recruitment, and it is powerful for women and employers alike to have these stories being told.

WORK180 is currently operating in Australia, the United Kingdom, and the United States.

➜ *Find out more at www.work180.com.*

CIRCLE IN

Circle In was founded by Jodi Geddes and Kate Pollard in Australia in 2017. The platform now services employees and employers across ten countries including Australia, New Zealand, the U.S., U.K., and Canada.

Circle In provides a personalized online employee benefits platform designed to offer support to working parents/families and carers, offering direct guidance for individual team members and providing useful tools and resources for managers who may not be trained in how to best support team members with caring responsibilities. The platform works alongside other HR resources, and is tailored to suit the needs of the organization. Circle In provides online resources that employees can access themselves, on topics relative to their unique needs as parents and carers. The platform is equipped to provide working parents, caregivers and managers with tools and resources aligned to each stage of parenthood, available anytime, anywhere.

Circle In is still a young company but in the four short years in which they have been operating, they have already achieved amazing success, having partnered with many companies globally (and achieving a 100 percent renewal rate amongst existing customers) and assisting over 200,000 families.

➜ https://circlein.com/

MEDIBANK

Medibank Private Limited is one of the largest Australian private health insurance providers and the organization employs approximately 4,000 people. In 2018, it became one of the first employers in Australia to remove the labels of 'primary' and 'secondary' carer in its parental leave policy providing that all employees, regardless of gender, can access the company's paid parental leave benefits of fourteen weeks' salary within the first twenty-four months of the birth or adoption of a baby[82]. The company made the change to improve equality within the organization and, as a result, has increased the percentage of its male employees taking parental leave from 2.5 percent to thirty percent.

➜ https://www.medibank.com.au/

---

82. https://www.medibank.com.au/livebetter/newsroom/post/medibank-rewrites-the-rules-parental-leave/

GIRLS WHO CODE

Girls Who Code is on a mission to close the gender gap in technology, and to change the image of what a programmer looks like, and does. It is a nonprofit organization which aims to support and increase the number of women in computer science by equipping young women with the necessary computing skills to pursue twenty-first century opportunities.

Girls Who Code provide programs and internships to women in technology, and they partner with companies to support the expansion of opportunities for women in technology across the world.

→ *https://girlswhocode.com/*

MEESHO

Meesho, is an Indian social e-commerce company, headquartered in Bangalore, India. In September 2021, the company announced its new thirty-week gender-neutral parental leave policy which applies equally to women, men, heterogenous or same-sex couples. Employees are eligible for leave of up to one year with thirty weeks fully paid leave, and twenty-five percent pay for the next three months. The policy also applies to the company's employees whether they have children born naturally, through surrogacy or through adoption. Meesho's policy aims to ensure non-discriminatory benefits, irrespective of employee's gender or sexual identity.

→ https://meesho.com/

WOMEN'S AGENDA

Women's Agenda is an Australian-based platform which shares the latest news and views affecting how women live and work. Women's Agenda is published by the 100 percent female-owned and run Agenda Media. Their team of journalists publish news stories on current affairs, political issues impacting women, women's health, women in business, leadership, workplace issues, the climate, life, and events. Women's Agenda also has its own podcast called The Women's Agenda Podcast[83].

---

83. https://womensagenda.com.au/podcasts/

Women's Agenda is a fantastic news source of current issues impacting women across the globe. I read their articles every day and I am constantly saving links to their webpages or taking screenshots of their stories. I highly recommend following this platform and their journalists.

→ https://womensagenda.com.au/

PARENTS@WORK

Parents@Work is a workplace culture and coaching organization. Since 2014, the company has been providing coaching for working parents. Parents@Work enables companies to build up their own peer coaching program for parents, using existing resources – upskilling employees with coaching skills and equipping future leaders with new perspectives and increased empathy, with the aim of creating family friendly workplace cultures so that parents can achieve their full potential at work.

→ https://www.parentsatwork.com/

CARROT

Carrot is a global fertility benefits provider, managing employee fertility benefits programs on behalf of employers. Carrot helps employers to offer their employees fertility benefits that are flexible, transparent, cost-conscious and legally compliant in each jurisdiction where they service employees and employers. Carrot is a complete and modern solution for those employers that are looking to provide benefits programs that are outside the norm, and there is clearly much demand for their services because they have just managed to raise USD $75 million in a series C round capital raise[84].

There is no doubt that Carrot has found a gap in the employee benefits market and as someone who personally had to use fertility treatments myself, I very much welcome these initiatives and would encourage more employers to consider implementing fertility benefits. To an employee that is experiencing challenges

---

84. https://www.forbes.com/sites/rebeccaszkutak/2021/08/17/fertility-startup-carrot-raises-75-million-in-a-series-c-round-led-by-tiger-global/?sh=407852204218

conceiving, and members of the LGBTQ+ community, fertility benefits can be more valuable than any salary that a company can offer.

→ https://www.get-carrot.com/

KIDSCO

KidsCo is an Australian organization that is assisting parents with what has become a fundamental need as a result of COVID-19 – planning, organizing and facilitating virtual educational fun when parents have to work, and onsite support during school holidays. KidsCo partners with employers to provide employees with access to their virtual services – which can range from short sessions after school to full day sessions during school holiday periods. The child can be in the same room as the employee or in the room next to them, but the employee has the support needed to continue their job in the knowledge that their child is not only being occupied but he or she is also learning.

→ https://www.kidsco.net.au/

BRIGHT HORIZONS

Bright Horizons is a childcare provider that operates in a number of countries. They provide onsite childcare services both for more permanent placements and on an as-needed basis. They also provide a service called back-up care, which can be accessed when nannies cancel, during school closures or school holidays for example. Bright Horizons partners with employers to customize a tailored solution for each company and their employees, and the services can be accessed and booked through an app. It is a fantastic program and one that I can personally highly recommend as we are extremely fortunate to have this benefit for all of our staff at my firm, Littler. When my twins were younger and I was travelling frequently for work, I would often take them with me. I was able to use the back-up care services to arrange childcare for my twins when I had meetings to attend in different cities around the world. Bright Horizons can also provide virtual childcare and education support, and they run events and education sessions for parents on various family, childcare, and schooling issues.

→ https://www.brighthorizons.com/family-solutions/back-up-care

BUSINESS CHICKS

With the super-impressive entrepreneur and author Emma Isaacs at the helm, Business Chicks has become a successful and globally recognized business and professional community of like-minded women, aimed at providing members and those who attend their events, workshops, conferences or retreats with the tools needed to propel individuals and businesses forward. The Business Chicks community is welcoming and full of interesting, intelligent, and highly successful women. Their events are first-class, full of fun, and there is just something extremely special about this organization, which is why so many companies are supporters. They offer many ways for employers to get involved – including through group memberships for employees. I have probably attended close to 100 Business Chicks webinars, conferences, events and retreats, and I have also presented a workshop on U.S. market entry for members. Business Chicks provides women with a supportive environment where they can share challenges and successes with other women, creating a professional network that can assist a person throughout their career. Many of the members will support the businesses of other members where they can and through COVID-19 many donated products, services, and money to assist those members who have struggled as a result of the repeated lockdowns in Australia. I highly recommend considering memberships for your employees in this great organization or sending your employees to one of their events.

→ https://businesschicks.com/about-us/

MEGAPORT LTD

I couldn't include a chapter about what innovative companies around the world are doing to better assist women in the workplace without talking about one of my own organizations, Megaport Limited. I am incredibly proud of the organization and the initiatives that we have implemented to date, and they are proving successful as we have managed to continue to improve our gender diversity profile within the employee population, on the executive team and on our board. We are now at fifty/fifty men and women on the board.

As a technology company, we recognize that we have a role to play in the achievement of equality within the technology industry as, like most technology companies, we too have traditionally been a heavily male-dominated organization – but that is changing through the continued efforts of our leadership.

Some of the benefits that we have implemented for our employees globally include the following:

- Twelve weeks company paid parental leave for men and women – no primary or secondary carer distinction
- Vacation leave purchase policy
- Five days paid miscarriage leave per occasion
- Continuation of paid employee retirement benefits during unpaid parental leave periods
- Five days paid emergency leave in situations of personal emergency or to provide care or support for a member of the employee's family
- $5,000 study allowance for an approved course
- Paid birthday leave
- EAP services
- Employee annual share allotment.

➔ https://www.megaport.com/

WOMEN RISING & MICROSOFT

Women Rising, which was founded by CEO Megan Dalla-Camina, and Microsoft have partnered together to create the Women Rising program, which is a six-month virtual program that offers women expert coaching to build their career plan and personal brand. The program is available to women at all levels and there is also an additional leadership program, Women Rising Manager Program. The course contains eight modules that cover vision and purpose, radical confidence, career evolution, authentic leadership, influence and impact, intentional wellbeing, grit and grace and leading change. The Women Rising program aims to support women in business to become confident, authentic leaders and the Women Rising Manager Program aims to support managers to become better mentors, sponsors and allies for other women.

➔ https://www.womenrisingco.com/

FORBES WOMEN

Forbes Women is a division of the U.S. business magazine. Forbes Women covers news on current affairs, political issues impacting women, women's health, women in business, leadership, and workplace issues.

Forbes Women is another great source of news regarding issues impacting women and they regularly highlight successful women across the globe.

→ https://www.forbes.com/forbeswomen/

HEADSPACE FOR WORK

Headspace for Work is a science-backed meditation and mindfulness solution for the workplace. Headspace for Work sells bundled subscriptions of their popular meditation app to companies worldwide, boasting a simple but important promise to employers, *Happier people. Healthier business.*

Headspace for Work also offers employers the ability to manage and see the impact of the program on their employees through the employer dashboard, engagement resources and measurement tools.

→ https://www.headspace.com/work

THRIVE GLOBAL

Thrive Global is the brainchild of Huffington Post founder, Arianna Huffington. As the statement on their website says, "Employee Well-being is No Longer a Benefit. It's a Strategy." They aim to assist companies to better manage employee stress and burnout by providing change technology and tools to assist people to live and work with less stress, so that they can be more productive and experience greater wellbeing. Thrive Global offers an app, micro learning programs, live webinars, and stories of leadership journeys as well as custom insights and analytics.

→ https://thriveglobal.com/

WOMEN'S TECH FORUM

The Women's Tech Forum is an organization that is focused on connecting women in the cloud, networking, and data center infrastructure industry. The origin of the organization's story came from asking two simple questions:"Why aren't there more women in our industry?" and "How come more of us don't know each other?"

Women's Tech Forum is focused on connecting women in tech, providing resources, education, and events.

→ https://www.womenstechforum.com/

NETFLIX

The streaming platform Netflix needs no introduction, but they have become famous for other reasons outside the great shows that they have produced. Netflix offers the longest paid family leave by far out of all the tech companies, and indeed, their parental leave benefit is far more generous than more other companies globally. In 2018, the company announced that all salaried employees, including birth and adoptive parents of any gender, can take up to a year off at full pay following the birth or adoption of their child. Later, the company extended its parental leave benefit to all of its employees. Hourly employees are entitled to between twelve and sixteen weeks of paid leave, depending on their position/department.

Netflix also offers a number of additional, generous employee benefits, including unlimited vacation days for salaried employees.

→ https://www.netflix.com/

MYOB

MYOB is one company that is leading the way on issues impacting women in the workplace. The tax, accounting and business services software company has been vocal about fostering a culture to better support its women at work, including through workplace flexibility, providing childcare support, implementing better digital support for their employees to log on and keep on top of their work while being with their kids, and through educating and training managers to lead by example and manage their employees in a more supportive and inclusive way[85]. The company has been a big proponent of motivating staff with the right employee benefits, as they recognize the link to

---

85. https://www.myob.com/au/blog/how-business-can-support-working-mums/

productivity and employee retention[86]. MYOB releases blog posts on many issues related to workplace equality and employee benefits which can be found on its website.

→ https://www.myob.com/au

JOHNSON & JOHNSON

Johnson & Johnson is a household name across many parts of the globe. It is also an organization that has been thinking up and implementing ways to better support its employees for over thirty years and is a trailblazer on employee wellness initiatives and benefits. Even as far back as the late 1970s Johnson & Johnson had recognized the importance of wellbeing and created a culture of health.

The company has conducted its own research over the years and has indicated that its wellness programs have been a wise investment. The company's own research has showed that every dollar it spends on wellness programs yielded a potential $2 to $4 return on investment.

Since 1995, the percentage of Johnson & Johnson employees who smoke has dropped by more than two-thirds. The number who have high blood pressure or who are physically inactive also has declined by more than half.

Additionally, Johnson & Johnson is one of the U.S. Corporations that have joined together with others including Coca-Cola Co., Verizon Communications, Inc., Bank of America Corp., Walgreen Co., McKinsey & Co., Blue Cross and Blue Shield Association, Aetna Inc. and Advanced Health Combined to form a group called the CEO Council on Health and Innovation which aims to improve employee and community health and reduce costs. Several council members have initiated uccessful wellness initiatives within their own companies and are encouraging other companies to follow suit.

Some of the other employee benefits that the company provides include:

- Adoption (up to $20,000), fertility (up to $35,000) and surrogacy benefits (up to $20,000)

---

86. https://www.myob.com/au/blog/offering-the-right-employee-benefits/

- Pet insurance
- Full salary for up to twenty-four months for employees enlisted in the military and called to active duty
- Global paid parental leave
- Energy for Performance® courses
- Breast milk shipping
- Extended volunteer leave policy
- Onsite and subsidized childcare benefits
- Medical and surgical coverage and support for employees diagnosed with gender dysphoria
- Special needs assistance through Bright Horizons
- College coaching for employees and their children
- Paid new father days.

→ https://www.jnj.com/

PEPSICO

PepsiCo is another company that needs no introduction, but it too has a long history of employee benefits and wellness initiatives which are aimed to better assist employees, and importantly, women within the workplace. Through their own research, they have documented positive results, cost savings and significant return on investment as a result of these initiatives. Some of the employee benefits that the company provides include:

- Life insurance
- Legal assistance
- Healthy living programs
- Healthy money programs
- Retirement benefit matching
- Paid parental leave
- Adoption assistance
- Paid child and elder care leave
- Scholarship program for children
- Tuition reimbursement for employees
- Paid medical, dental and vision insurance benefits.

→ https://www.pepsico.com/

ENDOMETRIOSIS AUSTRALIA

Founded by Donna Ciccia and Jodie Dunne in 2012, Endometriosis Australia is a not-for-profit organization in Australia that is focused on endometriosis awareness, support and research. The organization provides education programs and, through fundraising initiatives, helps to fund endometriosis research. Endometriosis Australia also creates and provides professional, educational programs for women with endometriosis, communities, schools, healthcare professionals and businesses. As endometriosis is a disease that impacts so many women globally, it is something that has the potential to impact every single employer. Awareness about the disease and its debilitating symptoms, and how they can impact a woman at work is step one, but more funding to support research into better diagnosis and treatment options are also badly needed.

To find out more about how you can help or to donate, please go to the Endometriosis Australia website:

→ https://www.endometriosisaustralia.org/how-can-you-help
→ https://www.endometriosisaustralia.org/

SURROGACY AUSTRALIA

Surrogacy Australia is another organization that I am involved with. I am one of the organization's non-executive directors and am responsible for corporate relations.

Surrogacy Australia fulfills an important role in Australia by providing information and support to people who are planning to be, or who are already parents via surrogacy arrangements. Surrogacy is a complex issue, and the law can vary significantly from one state or country to the next. Surrogacy Australia works with politicians, academics, and the media to educate, dispel myths and lobby for laws to protect surrogates, intended parents and children.

One of the other services that Surrogacy Australia provides employers, is employee surrogacy information and support service programs. The organization is able to tailor a program specific to an organization and its employees which can include information, introductions to surrogacy lawyers, fertility doctors, counselling services and connection to a network of other surrogates and families that have children that were born via a surrogacy arrangement.

→ https://www.surrogacyaustralia.org/

THE HEALTH PROJECT

The Health Project, Inc. (The Health Project), is a tax-exempt not-for-profit corporation formed to bring about critical attitudinal and behavioral changes addressing the health and well-being of Americans. The organization highlights employers that implement programs that have measurably improved the health and well-being of employees. They also award one company with the C. Everett Koop National Health Award each year to recognize outstanding worksite health promotion and improvement programs

→ http://thehealthproject.com/year/2020/

WOMEN ON BOARDS

Women On Boards is an organization that describes itself as a "league of extraordinary women". Women on Boards has been working since 2006 to address gender inequity in the boardroom and across leadership roles through events, programs, networking, support services, mentoring opportunities and access to information. Upon joining, members are provided with:

- Access to leadership and development programs and opportunities
- Better ability to understand and talk about your transferable skills
- A template for a board-ready CV and knowledge of what you bring to the table
- A strategic framework for getting a board role – now and in the future
- Access to a wide range of board positions
- Access to their members only online community – WOBShare.

→ https://www.womenonboards.net/

WOMEN IN THE BOARDROOM

Women in the Boardroom is an organization that is focused on assisting women to obtain board positions. They offer programs such as Matchmaking Program®, Annual Board Assembly and networking events and webinars as well as courses and board strategy services to organizations, including to those that are looking to improve diversity within their organizations.

→ https://womenintheboardroom.com/

WORKPLACE GENDER EQUALITY AGENCY

The Workplace Gender Equality Agency is an Australian Government statutory agency that promotes and improves workplace gender equality, and administers the Workplace Gender Equality Act 2012 (Act). The agency is responsible for overseeing the mandatory compliance reporting on gender equality that applies to all employers in Australia with 100 or more employees.

The agency also provides employers with access to useful information related to gender equality and issues impacting women at work. It also provides an opportunity for employers in Australia to receive Employer of Choice status for gender equality[87]. Important criteria that must be met in order to achieve the accreditation include:

- Leadership, strategy, and accountability
- Developing a gender-balanced workforce
- Gender pay equity
- Support for carers
- Mainstreaming flexible work
- Preventing gender-based harassment and discrimination, sexual harassment, and bullying
- Driving change beyond your workplace.

→ https://www.wgea.gov.au/

FUTURE SUPER

Future Super is an Australian superannuation fund (retirement benefit provider) that in February 2021 implemented a menstrual and menopause leave policy which provides employees with an additional six days of paid leave per year on top of their regular personal leave entitlements in situations where they

---

87. https://www.wgea.gov.au/what-we-do/employer-of-choice-for-gender-equality

are experiencing illness or severe symptoms associated with menstruation, menopause, or related health conditions. The policy was implemented after consideration for the impact symptoms of menstruation and menopause can have on the organization's female employees, and to remove related stigma and taboo as part of a larger vision for equality within each organization. The policy was designed and implemented in partnership with the Victorian Women's Trust. Future Super also have a collaborative group within their organization dedicated to equality, called SuperGenders. "SuperGenders aims to share experiences and ideas to improve Future Super, as well as support and celebrate gender diversity and inclusion both personally and professionally."[88]

➜ https://www.futuresuper.com.au/

GAZOOP

Gazoop is a digital communications agency company in India that first introduced an employee menstrual leave policy in 2017. The company's policy states that women may work from home one day per month during menstruation. The company has essentially explained that they want women to work from the comfort of their homes, be able to do so on comfortable chairs in their own environments and remove any stress associated with menstruation and work. They have also reiterated that this does not make the gender less hireable[89]. About seventy-six percent of the female workforce have used their menstrual leave since implementation. The Gazoop policy differs from other menstrual leave policies in that it offers workplace flexibility instead of leave.

➜ https://www.gozoop.com/

ACCENTURE

Multinational professional services company Accenture offers flexibility to its employees by empowering them to choose how, when and where they work.

---

88. https://www.futuresuper.com.au/blog/a-bloody-good-policy/

89. https://www.mansworldindia.com/uncategorized/in-conversation-with-the-pioneers-who-have-implemented-menstrual-leave-policy-in-their-organisations/

The company also has an app-based Accenture Active initiative. It encourages employees to choose a key wellness goal that matters to them and then supports and rewards them for accomplishing it.

Accenture places a major emphasis on the mental wellbeing of its staff. There's an appreciation at the company that, sometimes, work-related stress can be linked closely to what's going on outside the workplace. There are confidential support services available to help employees with issues like stress, substance abuse, depression, and anxiety as well.

→ https://www.accenture.com/

COEXIST FOUNDATION

Coexist Foundation, a social enterprise organization in the U.K., offers their female workers the option of one paid day of menstrual leave per month. Bex Baxter, Coexist's former People Development Manager, dealt with dysmenorrhea for years before developing a flexible menstrual leave policy that would support Coexist's female staff. The following statement appears on the organization's website about Coexist's policy: "Menstruating staff who opt into the policy are entrusted to respect their cycle and take responsibility for their own well-being... they need to check in with their line manager regarding their individual well-being requirements, and in any instance, any time off or alteration to their working hours must be communicated and signed off with their manager. Some roles allow menstruating staff the option to work from home, or alternatively to use a quiet space away from the main office... Coexist recognizes the importance of difference and debate, therefore should an employee not wish to take part in the policy, they can request to opt out with no judgement or discussion."

Coexist also offers all of their employees 'well-being rooms' where menstruators and non-menstruators alike can take a moment to focus on their health and wellness during work hours.

→ https://www.coexistfoundation.org/

CULTURE AMP

Founded in 2009, Culture Amp is an employee engagement, performance management and development platform headquartered in San Francisco although it has offices and employees across the world. The organization aims to assist businesses to transform and build a competitive advantage by putting culture first. In 2021, Culture Amp was named to Fast Company's annual list of the World's Most Innovative Companies[90].

Culture Amp's annual conference – Culture First – brings together its community members and connects people to share perspectives, ideas, advice, and information on assisting people to grow and thrive at work through creating an inclusive culture. The Culture Amp website contains a wealth of useful information on People Science, and how to pinpoint and resolve an organization's culture challenges with the latest research and expert guidance. This includes research and data science from the world's largest collection of employee insights and benchmarking across demographics, industries and more. A lot of this information is available free for anyone to access, and the organization also has its own podcast, *Culture First, Stories from a journey in building a better world of work*[91]. Culture Amp is a company to watch.

➜ https://www.cultureamp.com/

WORKDAY

Workday, Inc., is U.S. headquartered ondemand financial management and human capital management software company that operates across more than thirty countries. In addition to offering workplace flexibility, Workday provides various employee benefits that include sports teams, Dogs@Workday, cantinas, fitness and yoga, family events, employee stock plans, commuter programs, health plans, back-up childcare, car wash, discount tickets, vehicle maintenance, dry cleaning, hair salon, health assessments, healthy

---

90.   https://www.cultureamp.com/company/announcements/culture-amp-named-to-fast-companys-annual-list-of-the-worlds-most-innovative-companies-for-2021

91. https://www.cultureamp.com/podcast?season=1

food options, annual flu shots, banking and monthly chair massages. Workday has also implemented an Elevate program where C-Suite livestream events cover topics from "The Changing World of HR" to an interview with Usain Bolt. Through the Elevate platform, Workday interviews thought leaders and executives across the world as they share their stories of leading change, sharing the highs and lows from the front-line of business transformation.

→ http://www.workday.com/

INTUIT

Intuit Inc. is financial software company based in the U.S., but with offices across the world. The organization has established the Intuit Women's Network for female power to prosper at Intuit by helping women to #BalanceForBetter[92]. Through the network, the organization invests and supports women through various initiatives. It also celebrates "amazing game changing women". As Intuit highlights, "Gender balance is not only a social issue, but it also affects businesses and productivity. At Intuit we believe it's important to support and champion all women and especially women in fields such as STEM, where the balance of male to female technologists is still heavily skewed male." Through the network, Intuit aims to find ways to support its employees and enhance their skills through career development initiatives.

→ https://www.intuit.com/

LEAN IN

Lean In is a global community dedicated to helping women achieve their ambitions and work to create an equal world. Through the platform, Lean In has assisted more than 50,000 women in 184 countries to start Lean in Circles, which are communities of women who join together in a safe space to share struggles, give and get advice and celebrate each other's wins[93].

---

92. https://www.intuit.com/blog/intuitlife/international-womens-day-intuit-womens-network-helps-balanceforbetter/
93. https://leanin.org/circles

Lean In's Co-Founder and Board Chair, Sheryl Sandberg (CFO of Facebook) created Lean In after writing her book of the same name as she believes that "We need more women at every table where decisions are made. We need to push back against gender inequality in every form – now more than ever."

Lean In offers a company partner program where the organization can help companies to close the gender leadership gap within their own organizations and connect like-minded companies together in a community to share and access data, training materials, HR practices, benchmarking, and to track progress. The organization also offers a lot of free information and resources for employers on its website.

If you haven't read Sandberg's book *Lean In*, do yourself a favor a grab a copy!

→ https://leanin.org/

UN WOMEN

UN Women is the United Nations entity dedicated to gender equality and the empowerment of women. A global champion for women and girls, UN Women was established to accelerate progress on meeting their needs worldwide.

UN Women supports UN Member States as they set global standards for achieving gender equality and works with governments and civil society to design laws, policies, programs and services needed to ensure that the standards are effectively implemented and truly benefit women and girls worldwide.

UN Women provide useful training, resources, data and news and events that can be accessed and used by any employer.

→ https://www.unwomen.org/en

ASOS

Online fashion retailed Asos introduced a number of employee benefits in October 2021 including a policy to allow employees to work flexibly, as well as take time off at short notice, while going through the menopause, paid leave for staff who have experienced a pregnancy loss or are undergoing fertility treatment, with five days paid leave provided per cycle to ensure appointments can be attended. The company also now allows employees who are dealing with pregnancy loss, including miscarriages and abortions, to take 10 days of leave and employees with pregnant partners or those with children born via surrogate are also entitled to 10 days paid leave.

→ https://www.asos.com/

KELLOGG'S

Food manufacturer Kellogg's announced a range of new benefits in October 2021 including providing its employees with menopause, pregnancy loss and fertility treatment support, leave and financial assistance. The Company also announced plans to train its manager on how to talk about menopause and pregnancy loss with their employees so that better support and assistance can be provided.

→ https://www.kelloggcompany.com

While the companies embracing these new policies, programs and initiatives remain the exception, rather than the norm, they are nonetheless the innovators. They are good examples of organizations that are leading the way on employee wellness, and they are providing us with valuable data on the effectiveness of the various initiatives. Will every single one of them work? Probably not, and that is okay. The important thing is that they are businesses that recognize the human element in the workplace, they have recognized that finding ways to better support employees is a link to healthier and happier employees that are more productive, and they are actively taking steps to grow their awareness and strive for improvement. They have discovered this competitive edge, and they are examples that we should all be watching closely to learn from, adapt as needed and replicate within own organizations.

So, What Can You Do?

One of the things I get asked a lot is, "So, what can we do?" It's an important question. After all, the first step is acknowledgement, but the second critical step is to take action. Action starts with understanding – understanding about the status quo within your organization – because if you don't have a good sense of the existing lay of the land, then you cannot begin to effectively assess what might need to change. So, my advice would be, to analyze your culture, your systems, processes, salaries, and benefits, policies, and other workplace initiatives. Once you get a good sense of what currently exists you will have the foundation from which to get started.

The second thing I believe is critical to the development and implementation of an effective strategy for change, is communication with your people. As I have outlined throughout this book, there are many ways to achieve this, but regardless of how you decide to do it, it is crucial to hear from your employees because you need to know:

- Who are your employees?
- What are their struggles?
- What is important to them?
- Do they feel supported and able to share?
- What challenges do they face?
- What issues do they experience at work?
- What do they think could assist them?
- What are they looking for in their career/their employer?
- What benefits do they utilize and why?
- What benefits do they not use and why?
- What benefits would they like to see?
- What benefits are important to them?
- What type of flexibility, if any, are they seeking?
- What improvements do they think could be made to the workplace environment?
- What do your employees really care about when it comes to work?

When you are armed with this information, you will have a much better picture of the composition of your workforce and their struggles, experiences and needs at work. It should also provide you with some additional insights as well. For example, you might be an organization that is lacking in diversity, in which case you might not only need to listen to the needs of your existing employees, but also do some research on ways that you can try to attract more diverse candidates. This is something that we considered at Megaport. We knew that many of our existing employees were young men who may not be at a stage in their lives where they would need to access parental leave benefits, for example. What we also knew though, was that we wanted to attract more women to join the organization, and so we had to consider and anticipate what the needs of those employees that we were hoping to attract might be as well.

Think more creatively about employee benefits and workplace wellness initiatives. When we hear the term 'workplace wellness,' most people think about health sessions related to fitness, smoking, diet, or weight loss. However, workplace wellness actually means so much more. Many of these types of programs are also focused on fixing existing problems rather than preventing illness and injury, and promoting health and wellness generally. Program impacts are also not well-understood, and are often met with skepticism where the results may not be easily measurable. Try to think about how you will measure the true performance and value of any benefits programs or wellness initiatives that you might implement, in a much broader way.

Do your research and plan your business case. Boards want facts and they love data. Whether you are presenting to a board or not, plan as if you are and develop your business case. Utilize the research that I have outlined in this book and do your own research by scrolling through company websites and talking to other HR professionals about what has worked and not worked within their own organizations.

Ask them questions about the costs to the organization, whether they have any contacts or resources that they can share with you, and what the uptake and employee feedback has been since they introduced the benefit. Be realistic about the numbers. Set out a plan.

Don't expect a 'yes' to everything you ask for on day one, but set out goals for the organization and a timeline for implementation, and ask your leaders to get on board and commit to those goals.

Change the narrative around people and the workplace. Educate your leaders about the importance of employee wellness and the workplace. Approach it as if it is a health and safety issue, because in many respects, it actually is!

Initiate wellbeing into leadership at every level of the organization – lead with a culture of inclusiveness and support from the top, starting with the board. Shout it from the rooftop. If you don't let employees know that you care through your actions, then they will not believe it and you will never change the culture through mere words. Support and encourage healthy behaviors and wellness at work – at all levels. Don't let your CEO work through nights, travel fifty weeks a year and never take vacations. This doesn't demonstrate a good example for your employees, and ultimately it sets a tone throughout the whole organization and sends a message about the lack of priority for your employees, and their health and safety.

Implement employee progression and career plans. Ask your employees about their own goals, aspirations and dreams, and then help them achieve them – whether it is by remaining within your organization, or assisting them to find a company that is better aligned with their goals. Sometimes employees that don't seem as though their heart is really in the work are not motivated because they are not where they want to be. That's okay – but it can explain a lot, and sometimes it is far better to help an employee to find their purpose and pursue their dreams than never ask the question and waste time wondering why they seem disconnected or disengaged.

In order to recruit and retain high-performing employees, people managers must develop a talent strategy within the framework of the evolving workforce and working environment. Your talent strategies should prioritize the needs of both your existing employees, and the talent that you want to try to attract – at all stages of a their careers. Keep in mind that the benefits that a thirty-year-old female might be looking for in a workplace might be very different to those that a woman in her fifties might find beneficial. Don't forget your employees at any stage in their careers, as it is important to try to find a good balance of benefits, policies and initiatives that will cater for everyone.

Keep records and educate managers and executives when there are changes in leadership. If Joan has been an employee for ten years but she is out on extended sick leave as a result of undergoing cancer treatment – and in that time the management team changes – don't forget Joan! As part of an effective HR management system and handover, Joan, and anyone else like her should not be forgotten. The incoming incumbent should not be told merely the facts: Joan started on X date and is currently on leave due to cancer treatment. Rather, they should be educated on Joan's history in the organization, the fact that she is a valued employee and that someone needs to take over the responsibility of regularly checking in with her to make sure that she knows that we care, and will continue to be supportive regardless of any personnel changes. Unfortunately, this rarely happens and all too often, employees in Joan's situation get forgotten and eventually moved along.

Educate your managers on how to effectively communicate with their employees when they raise health issues. This is critical to break down the stigma that is associated with many female-health issues, menstruation, miscarriage, and menopause. Train your managers to regularly communicate with their employees about their wellbeing and to do more than just a cursory check-in. Most people have a natural tendency when asked, "Are you okay?" to instantly respond, "Yes. I'm fine" or "I'm okay" and sometimes that will be far from the truth.

Instead of asking an employee, "Are you okay?" ask them what you can do to assist and support them and offer suggestions so that employees do not need to be put in the awkward situation of having to ask for specific help themselves. It is a much more effective way of opening the door to a discussion about the specific support that an employee might need. It is also important to recognize that what works for one employee in a particular situation may not work for another. A one-size-fits-all approach therefore does not work for this reason.

Be open to different ideas, listen, and try to be flexible in your approach where possible. Equally, employees too should be open to suggestions and willing to discuss options and alternatives. Speaking up brings with it a power of its own. Don't assume your employer doesn't want to help and support you just because they cannot accommodate your exact request. Sometimes it is simply not possible, but there might be another option that could work for both parties.

Prioritize your employee mental health, especially right now. A lot is said about Employee Assistance Programs (EAP) and whether they still have a place today. Some companies feel they are not effective because they are not widely utilized. I disagree. Much like myself, many people who are supporters of therapy, want consistency and someone they can build a relationship with over time, so these employees will often have their own therapist that they see regularly. I don't see the role of EAPs for this purpose though. EAP is really there to serve employees in times of crisis much like we are in right now as a result of the COVID-19 global pandemic.

EAPs are there to assist those employees who are not regular users of therapy. The hope is of course that no employee will feel the need to use the service. However, I do not believe that relatively small usage equals a failed or outdated benefit. Additionally, many of my clients have told me that through the COVID-19 they have seen their EAP usage significantly increase as more and more people are finding the need to talk to someone – with lockdowns, closed borders and travel restrictions continuing – which has meant that many are alone and without connection to colleagues, friends, and family. Having an existing EAP in place has been one more way for these companies to continue to assist and support their employees through an incredibly challenging period. If EAP is not for you though, find other ways to connect with, check-in on and support your employees with their mental health periodically, especially during difficult times.

Every single one of us is a leader within our own families, and our own communities. We all impact others through our decisions, words, actions, and choices. Leadership is a skill that every one of us needs to continue to work on and strive for improvement throughout our careers. Every person has the power to influence change within our own communities and when we witness inequality in the workplace, we all should be taking a stand. Importantly though, change starts first in the home. For those of us with children, grandchildren, nieces, nephews, or other young people in our lives, they are the future. They learn from our example. Make sure that they learn from our mistakes, and they enter the workforce with a different mindset – one where we strive to help others, where people are treated equally, and we respect one another. The best way of educating our young people is by leading by example. This is why things like mentoring and finding ways to share your experiences and offer advice to young people is so important.

WHAT I DID TO MAKE POSITIVE CHANGES IN MY OWN LIFE

We are all on life's journey and one of the best things we can do for ourselves is to invest time in our health and wellbeing. Whether your employer recognizes it or not, nothing is more important than your health. When our health is diminished, so too is our quality of life. It took me a long time to realize this and prioritize my own health. As I have explained to you throughout this book, I made a lot of mistakes, but I am almost sure that they are similar to the mistakes that so many of you are continuing to make today – not taking leave, not resting, pushing through, all for fear of the repercussions.

I understand that we are all living busy lives, and some are not in a position where they feel able to raise these types of issues with their employer. For those women, I will continue to speak out for you, and I hope that those of you that are in leadership positions will continue to do the same. However, there are still steps that every one of us can take to implement better self-care and wellness into our lives.

If it means getting up even twenty minutes earlier or going to bed twenty minutes later so that you can get that walk, run, or exercise program in, listen to a meditation or calming music on an

App like Calm[94] or read a book just for pleasure, schedule the time. Do it for yourself. The science proves that it works. The results of a new study published in August 2021, show that the exercise hormone irisin is a critical regulator of cognitive function[95]. Scientists have discovered that exercise may actually bolster brain health, including by altering the trajectory of memory loss. Wellness doesn't need to mean that you train for a marathon. It means taking time out to do something that is just for you.

It took me nine surgeries before I finally realized that the way that I was working, and living was not good for my body or my mind. As I continued to push through and I continued to get sick, I finally realized that something had to change. Was it not for the arrival of my daughters though, and the fact that they became my priority and my 'why', I wonder if I might never have made the changes that I did?

I would like to believe that I would have ended up here regardless, but I know how difficult it is to get stuck on the hamster wheel or feel like you are trapped in a situation where you are screaming silently for help, but no one can hear you. I know what it is like to desperately want to achieve at work so that you can get that promotion, but inside you are suffering in physical or emotional pain due to endometriosis or the loss of a baby. Or how difficult it is when work demands just don't allow for any human frailty, or so we believe. And, in those moments I know how hopeless and hard it all seems, and how far from your mind looking after your own health and wellness may be. But I also know there is only so far that you can continue to push before the system will fail, and that there really is a better way that leads to much more positive results, both personally and professionally.

For me, the only way I was finally able to take better care of myself was by learning to say no sometimes. This was essential as I set about defining the life I wanted, finding ways to create better balance in my life and coming to terms with the fact that I *could* have it all but not all at the same time! I began to work on setting better boundaries

94. https://www.calm.com/

95. https://www.nature.com/articles/s42255-021-00438-z

and more realistic expectations for my clients and presenting solutions to problems rather than just focusing on the issue; asking for help when needed and taking time off work when I was sick and allowing my body the time that it needed to heal and recover, even taking actual vacations where I spend time present with my family and without my devices. I began using apps such as Calm and Ten Percent Happier for relaxation and mediation and finding ways to regularly reflect and journal the things that I am grateful for, taking better control of my healthcare and doing more research to find better providers. I found time to integrate some Chinese medicine into my treatment and scheduled time in my calendar for fitness, the occasional massage and, of course, reading and writing!

These are just some of the things I did to improve my health, reduce the symptoms associated with my medical conditions, and implement better balance and happiness into my life and, as I have told you, once I did that, I started to see the benefits. I had an extremely successful year at work, since then I am a better mother and the time I spend with my children is more quality time. Plus, I have been able to serve on a number of boards doing work that I love, as well as write this book! That is something that I could simply not have achieved had I continued on the path I was on for so long.

In her 2021 book *Your Time to Thrive*, Arianna Huffington talks about making "micro steps" towards a healthier life to avoid stress and burnout. I would suggest that the same advice equally applies here. Small or micro steps all make a difference when it comes to wellness. It doesn't have to mean that you need to stop or even slow down, but I can assure you that if you keep going at inhuman speeds you will eventually be forced to do so!

Wellness is about finding better ways to be more productive when we are 'on' by looking after ourselves and switching 'off' sometimes, based on the needs of our bodies and minds, and what that looks like will be different for every person. I have given you all of my insights, ideas, beliefs and advice. It is up to each of you to take it on board and implement better practices within your own life. So, go out there and find your own way to thrive!

I would like to leave you with some ideas for organizations as well as some personal tips.

Just a Few Ideas....

- Health risk assessments/biometric Screenings including health risk assessments for cholesterol and blood pressure levels;
- Disease Management;
- Financial Counseling/Planning;
- Fitness Classes;
- Flexible Work Schedules;
- Flu Shots;
- Free Healthy Food;
- Gym Reimbursement;
- Health Coaching;
- Health Education;
- Health Fairs;
- On-Site Clinics;
- Telemedicine;
- Tobacco Cessation;
- Assistance with alcohol addiction;
- Weight Management;
- Wellness Challenges;
- Period policies including flexibility and leave;
- Menopause policies including flexibility;
- Financial counseling and planning;
- Fitness classes;
- Access to therapists or career coaches – more than just EAP;
- On-Demand childcare/back-up care;
- A 'benefits bank' where employees are allocated a certain value and they can select from a selection of options that suit them;
- Fertility benefits including IVF, surrogacy and adoption allowances and support services including counselling and access to agencies;
- Egg freezing;
- Miscarriage counseling and access to support groups;

- Online and back-up childcare and education options for employees working from and managing children at home;
- Address the distinct challenges of women of color;
- Foster a culture that supports and values all women;
- Provide paid family leave benefits to all employees equally – removing the primary and secondary carer distinctions allows women the option of returning to work sooner. It also encourages a more equal distribution of childcare responsibilities within families;
- Make work requirements more sustainable through better flexibility in how work can be performed;
- Provide better feedback and performance reviews with constructive feedback.
- Implement career goals and progression plans for employees – it amazes me how few companies actually do this, despite being aware of their employees' aspirations;
- Set goals that align with the work requirements, the goals of the organization and the career aspirations of the employee;
- Conduct a thorough analysis of work processes, policies, procedures, and requirements to actively eliminate gender biases – both overt and indirect
- Get better at communicating with your employees – listen to them and encourage them to voice their opinions;
- Take action when you do receive employee feedback. Don't ask for it and then fail to find ways to improve;
- Find ways to better support employees so that they do not need to choose financial stability and job security over their health and wellbeing;
- Provide private break areas, pods, or rooms to accommodate mental health breaks, breastfeeding or women experiencing symptoms associated with a health condition and consider including sanitary products, clothing (for example branded t-shirts and pants etc. in multiple sizes), wipes, fans, books, deodorant, snacks, drinks etc.;
- Paid natural therapies such as massage, acupuncture, cupping etc.;

- Vacation expense reimbursement;
- Free books/workplace library;
- Flexible hours;
- Vacation purchase policy where employees can purchase additional leave by sacrificing some of their salary;
- Career break leave;
- Tuition assistance;
- Contribution to medical costs for any illness;
- Provide employees with access to 'femtech' including devices and apps to help track fertility, ovulation, menopause, female-cancers etc.;
- Offer leadership and career development courses that are catered to women;
- Consider the impacts of workplace conditions, practices, and benefits on all of your employees. Try to step into their shoes and think about how a particular group of employees might be impacted. For example, menstruation leave has been met with mixed opinion. However, if offered, this type of leave can greatly assist gender queer/non-binary individuals and transmen who might feel an increased sense of safety being able to work from home. For example, because menstruation may be a time in which these individuals face increased amounts of transphobia and other types of gender discrimination, not just at work but as they travel to and from the workplace as well.

MY FINAL PERSONAL TIPS FOR EACH OF YOU:

- Try to prepare at least a week ahead, ideally two;
- Keep old-school notebooks with lists;
- Use whiteboards and calendars;
- Mark off achievements and keep a record – in the tough times it really helps to look back on your achievements to give yourself a boost;
- Make personal wellness a priority! I have realized that this is absolutely crucial. I am unfortunately not someone who loves

exercise although believe me I have tried. However, I get up every day and I push myself to make time to do something. Usually, it is about thirty minutes on my iFit treadmill and for me that has made a world of difference. I now find that I have more energy, I am definitely happier and healthier. On those occasions when I might slip, I don't reprimand myself. I tell myself that I'll get up tomorrow and do better;

- Find sponsors and mentors and then pay it forward and mentor others.
- Connect with other like-minded people;
- Continue to speak up and share your own story, particularly if you are a leader or manager. Sharing your own vulnerabilities creates trust and demonstrates to others that you understand what they might be going through. It provides an easy way to create connection with others;
- If you take one small step each day you <u>WILL</u> make a difference. It is easy to get disheartened or overwhelmed and think that your voice doesn't matter, the problem is too big or that you don't have the platform to have any impact on change happening, and I am here to tell you that is absolutely not true. If you are the mother of a daughter, you can start by having discussions with your daughter about these issues and setting examples. If you are the mother of a son, you can have a positive impact on future generations by teaching your son about why he should care about these issues, because he might be the next founder or leader of an organization and have the power to implement policies to assist women in the future;
- It takes inner strength to do what we need to do, so we need to support one another to have the confidence to raise our voice;
- Lead with compassion – show others that you genuinely care. Compassion at work leads to positive results both for individual wellbeing and for the organization as well as it creates trust, satisfaction, loyalty, and innovation
- Give constructive feedback;
- Encourage others to come up with solutions when presented with issues in the workplace. You attract more flies with honey

than with vinegar. I have certainly personally experienced this, and I have realized that when I flip the narrative and focus on solutions to a problem rather than the problem itself, it tends to generate a much more favorable response;

- Debrief with someone. For me, I do this through weekly sessions with my therapist. I value those sessions immensely and, in my opinion, everyone should do regular therapy. I am a huge advocate for this. Unfortunately, most people go to a therapist during times of crisis and stop once their lives return to some 'normality'. In my view that is a flawed approach. Going regularly means that I am much better prepared to deal with stressful situations as and when they arise. However, even if therapy is not for you, a life coach, a mentor or even just a friend who is a good listener, doesn't judge and is able to offer you support and love can provide a similar benefit;

- Remember to speak up for diversity, equality, and inclusion whenever you can, especially when it relates to the vulnerability of others who may not be in a position to do so. Diverse organizations are more productive and successful in many ways. Don't forget that;

- Don't just talk the talk. You have to walk the walk!

Closing

I never could have imagined the journey that my life would take me on. When I decided to move to the United States at the age of twenty-eight, I was escaping Australia, but I also looked at it as an amazing opportunity and the start of a new beginning. I now have a great understanding and appreciation for all that I have gone through in my life, and my journey is far from complete.

I have learnt a lot about society and culture and have experienced some very painful and tough lessons along the way. I am sharing my story in the hope that I might be able to ignite a movement – one that demands change. I want more CEOs, founders, directors, human resources professionals and employees to start thinking about some of the issues that I have highlighted throughout this book and my hope is that more of you will find the strength to start discussions within your own organizations, communities and at home with your families – because for real change to occur it needs to happen everywhere.

We need to set examples for our employees, our colleagues our friends and our children about why equality should matter to everyone and the role that every single one of us plays in this journey. It is up to us to take personal and professional action to make changes. We need leaders who inspire change because when women thrive, we all thrive. We need to lead with empathy, compassion, and self-awareness. We must equally lead with our hearts. Support one another. There is not enough support by women of other women. Be there for each other.

Nearly every time someone has heard my story, they almost always say, "You should write a book". So, here it is. This is my story. I hope you have found it worth the read, that I have left you thinking and that you will go out into your own part of this world and start some 'uncomfortable' conversations within your workplace and beyond.

Thank you for letting me share my story with you.

Acknowledgements

I always love reading the acknowledgments section of a book because it usually gives a little more insight into the author and the person that they are, as people tend to surround themselves with like-minded people. In my case, I certainly hope you will also think that is true, because the people that I want to acknowledge and thank are all wonderful people and I am so blessed to have had the benefit of their help, support, advice, and guidance throughout this journey.

Thank you to my two researchers, Kate Voss, and Alana Thomas. As someone who used to try to avoid doing legal research wherever possible, I was not keen on the idea of having to pull together all of the data that I would require to write this book – but thankfully you both came to my rescue! Jokes aside, the data you compiled for me was extremely useful, interesting and thought-provoking, and as I read through it all, it just confirmed for me that I was definitely on the right track with my ideas in this book. Thank you again for all of your hard work and assistance.

To my uncle Mervyn, I have always admired you. You have been an inspiration to me throughout my life because you are so hard-working and passionate about everything that you do. Thank you for your help through the book's editing process.

To my colleagues at Littler, thank you for ten amazing years and for taking a chance on an unknown Aussie lawyer. I have had an incredible career and I am so grateful for the experiences and opportunities. A special thanks to my good friend and colleague, Tahl Tyson who has been so supportive of my mission. Tahl organized with me the first Littler event that was focused on women's health issues and the workplace. We might have shocked a few people at that event with some of the menstruation graphics, but I still recall it as one of the best events that I have ever presented at, and people were streaming up to us later to tell us the same thing. Let's make sure that it isn't our last!

To my colleagues at Surrogacy Australia – thank you, thank you, thank you for continuing the good fight, for raising awareness, educating people on this issue, and continuing to advocate for change.

To my Megaport family, but most importantly to Bevan Slattery, you gave me my first chance at a board position, and I have loved every single minute of it. I am so proud of the things that we have achieved already, and the exciting part is that we are just getting started. Bevan, I have already learnt so much from you. You are an inspiration, and I am so glad that I sat next to you on that flight.

Thank you so much to the courageous women who so selflessly and bravely shared their stories and experiences with us so that we could share them with you. It is never an easy thing to share your story, but I am so thankful to each of you for being willing to do so in the hope that we might be able to help others.

To my girlfriends Sharon Favero, Andrea Hunolt, Sherrijon Gaspard, Charlotta Pettersson, Kerry Willemsen and Sinead Phelan, thank you for your love, support, and encouragement (and the wines!) throughout this process.

Thank you to Simon Strong, the super-talented photographer who did the imagery for my book and the amazing Olivia Brown for the design, thank you to both of you for helping me to bring my vision to life. It is exactly what I envisioned!

To my book coach, Jas Rawlinson (https://www.jasrawlinson.com), wow, what can I say?! Firstly, thank you for your help interviewing and putting together the stories of the women we have featured in the book. Secondly, I have loved every minute of working with you. You are such an amazing help. You have offered me assistance, advice, support, and encouragement along the way, and I could not have done this without you so, thank you a million times over!

To my mother and my nana, thank you for teaching me about the importance of kindness, love, and compassion above all. I hope I have made you proud. Mom, thank you for your help with the editing, and for not being too critical of my grammar! Thank you for the support and encouragement of my journey to motherhood, and the love and help you have always given to Dave and myself when we've needed hands-on assistance with Adaline and Savannah who adore you! A huge thanks also for always being such an open book about your lives. At times, when I was a teenager, I felt it embarrassing to hear, but I now know that it is absolutely the best way to allow yourself to heal. By sharing your own experiences, in turn, I have learned to share my own and understand and help others who might be going through similar situations. Were it not for your example, I might never have written this book.

And lastly, but definitely not least, thank you so much to my husband Dave and my children Savannah and Adaline. Dave, I literally could not have achieved this dream without you. I know that it has been tough at times as I have spent days, nights and many weekends focused on my computer, but I am so thankful to you for allowing me the space to get through the process. I also want to thank you for something else though and that is for jumping in headfirst with me on the crazy, emotional, difficult, and expensive journey to create our family. Not once did you ever hesitate along the way. You were there, right by my side as we navigated the heartache of losing babies, the endless doctors' appointments, hospital visits, surgeries, IVF and right through the difficult surrogacy process. I know that none of it was easy on you either and I am grateful for your strength and support during that time. Most of all though, I am thankful to you for you helping to create, love and nurture our little 'munchkins'.

Savi and Adi, there are no words that I could ever say to express how much I love you and just how much my heart ached for you when you were both merely my heart's dream. You are my greatest achievement, my greatest love, my everything. You are the best part of me and everything that I do is for you.

You truly are, My Story!

About Naomi

Naomi Seddon is an international lawyer, thought leader, author, and presenter on issues impacting women at work.

A qualified lawyer in three countries, Naomi has assisted over 400 companies with their global expansion and was named a top attorney in the United States by Legal 500. Naomi is also a non-executive director of ASX company, Megaport Ltd and Surrogacy Australia and Co-Chair of United States, an international arts organization.

Naomi is a true expat. Having grown up in Australia, Naomi moved to Los Angeles, where she has lived for the last twelve years apart from a twelve-month stint in London. When not in L.A., Naomi is regularly off traveling around the world to assist her clients. However, her favorite place to be, by far, is with her daughters Savannah and Adaline, her husband Dave and their rapidly growing house of fur children – including their two Yorkies, Coco and Cappuccino, their cat Sooki, four fish (unnamed), two guinea pigs and one miniature horse.

You can connect with, or follow Naomi at:
- www.naomiseddon.com/ where you can sign up for updates and further book release information
- LinkedIn at https://www.linkedin.com/in/naomi-seddon-98b33433/
- Instagram @milkandmargaritas

NAOMI SEDDON - MILK & MARGARITAS

Work With Me

Are you an employer, company director, HR or people team professional who would like to know more about how you can implement positive changes within your organization to assist women? If so, I would love to assist you. For further information you can reach me at info@naomiseddon.com or through my website at www.naomiseddon.com/

Endometriosis Australia

Naomi is donating a percentage of the proceeds from the sale of Milk and Margaritas to Endometriosis Australia to assist the great work the organization is doing on raising awareness of the disease and furthering research into diagnosis and treatment options for all women.

You can find out more or donate here: https://www.endometriosisaustralia.org/